# WHY TAI CHI?

## QUESTIONS & ANSWERS
### MASTER C.K. CHU

*Edited by*
*Jeremy W. Hubbell, Ph.D.*

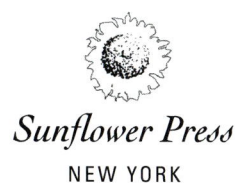

*Sunflower Press*
NEW YORK

Copyright © 2011 C.K. Chu

All rights reserved.

No part of this book may be used or reproduced in any manner whatsoever without written permission of the author.

Published by Sunflower Press
P.O. Box 750733, Forest Hills Station, NY 11375

Distributed by CK Chu Tai Chi
156 West 44th Street, New York, NY 10036
www.chutaichi.com

Why Tai Chi?
ISBN: 978-0-9832659-9-3
Library of Congress Control Number: 2011920387

First Edition

FOR STEPHANIE

# ACKNOWLEDGEMENTS

This book has been in my thoughts for a very long time, almost as long as I have been teaching and answering questions about tai chi. Many people, therefore, have contributed to the thinking behind this text. So to all of my students of the last four decades, thank you.

In the early 1990s, we published a journal called Peach Banquet which contained some Q&A. That, plus some other material made up the first version of this book but it was far more esoteric than the how-to approach needed when teaching tai chi. We renewed the effort with a new journal, Q&A by Master Chu in 2006, which is still in publication. Material generated in that effort became the nucleus of the present text. A few students were instrumental in asking questions and reviewing answers, including Jesse Shadoan, Hyland Harris, Nathaniel Wice, and Dan Zegibe. A special thanks to my writing assistant at the beginning, Dimitri Ehrlich. Aaron Bergeron also helped me with much of the writing and assembling of the text.

A special word of thanks to Jeremy W. Hubbell for finalizing the material to make it a book. The task was immense, though it doesn't seem like it. Answering questions thoroughly about tai chi is not a simple task. I am fortunate to have had his help finishing this book. He is hard working and he was extremely helpful in ironing out the content and seeing this book through to the end. Without him, the book might have taken another 20 years.

Hyland and Jesse helped with the photo section and Elizabeth Sharpe, my daughter, designed the cover and set the layout of the book.

Dolores Perin gave timely, valuable proofing and editing suggestions on the manuscript. A thank you to Jeremy R. Simon and Lidija Milic for their help with proofing the final manuscript. As always, my wife Carol was unyielding in her support and help in all stages of production.

This book would not have been produced without financial support. Thank you to the many people who donated during our 2010-2011 Pledge Drive especially our Platinum Level Contributors, Dan Nash and Dan Zegibe.

ALSO BY C.K.CHU

*Tai Chi Chuan Principles & Practice*

*The Book of Nei Kung*

*Chu Meditation*

*Eternal Spring Chi Kung*

# TABLE OF CONTENTS

| | |
|---|---|
| Note on this text | xv |
| Foreword: The Story of CK and Chu Tai Chi | xvii |
| Introduction | 1 |
| Tai Chi is a Fighting Art | 1 |
| Tai Chi is Science, Art, and Philosophy | 2 |
| Western Exercise | 3 |
| This Book | 5 |

## I. WHAT IS TAI CHI?

| | | |
|---|---|---|
| 1.1 | What is tai chi chuan? | 7 |
| 1.2 | What is the origin of tai chi? | 7 |
| 1.3 | How does tai chi differ from other Chinese martial arts? | 8 |
| 1.4 | What is the difference between tai chi and the other internal arts? | 9 |
| 1.5 | What is Taoism? | 9 |
| 1.6 | Is Taoism a religion? | 10 |
| 1.7 | What kind of Taoist are you? | 10 |
| 1.8 | What is the relationship between Taoism and tai chi? | 11 |
| 1.9 | So, is tai chi standardized? | 11 |
| 1.10 | Is Yang the most popular style because it is the easiest to learn? | 12 |
| 1.11 | Has tai chi been refined over the years? | 12 |
| 1.12 | What are the tai chi classics? Is the *Tao Te Ching* a tai chi classic? | 12 |
| 1.13 | What is tai chi's place in the history of martial arts? | 13 |
| 1.14 | When did tai chi come to the United States? Who brought it? | 13 |
| 1.15 | What does "lineage" mean in martial arts? | 14 |
| 1.16 | What is your lineage? | 14 |
| 1.17 | How does a Taoist school differ from a karate school? | 16 |
| 1.18 | What is the correct curriculum of tai chi chuan? | 16 |

## II. TAI CHI & HEALTH

| | | |
|---|---|---|
| 2.1 | What is the definition of health in your view? | 18 |
| 2.2 | How can tai chi help me achieve good health? | 18 |
| 2.3 | Why should I do tai chi instead of some other "maintenance" program? | 19 |
| 2.4 | What is *chi*? | 20 |
| 2.5 | Can the amount of *chi* be measured? | 21 |
| 2.6 | Could you elaborate on the role of *chi* in the body — the way it works, how it becomes obstructed, and how tai chi improves *chi* in the body? | 21 |
| 2.7 | What is alignment and why is it so important? | 22 |
| 2.8 | Is tai chi good for people with back and knee problems? | 23 |
| 2.9 | What is the importance of flexibility and coordination to health? | 24 |
| 2.10 | What effect does tai chi, *chi kung*, and *nei kung*, have on the body? | 25 |
| 2.12 | What is the problem with sports-based exercise? | 25 |
| 2.13 | How does running compare with tai chi? | 26 |
| 2.14 | What about weightlifting? | 26 |
| 2.15 | Besides using light weights, what are some exercises other than tai chi for strengthening the body? | 27 |
| 2.16 | Does Yoga deliver benefits similar to tai chi? | 27 |
| 2.17 | Is it true that tai chi slows the aging process? | 28 |
| 2.18 | What are your views about consumption of supplements, medicine, and stimulants (especially alcohol or other chemicals, either prescribed or not)? | 28 |
| 2.19 | On page 84 of *Tai Chi Chuan Principles & Practice* you discuss postnatal and prenatal breathing. What is the difference between the two? | 29 |
| 2.20 | What is the *tan tien* and what role, if any, does it have in tai chi? | 30 |
| 2.21 | Do we get a good cardiovascular workout from tai chi? | 30 |
| 2.22 | Can you elaborate on how slow and fast tai chi affect bodily systems? | 31 |
| 2.23 | Can you elaborate on the benefits of doing the tai chi form slowly? | 31 |
| 2.24 | So, does *wu wei* mean I can do the form however I want? | 32 |
| 2.25 | But how does relaxation come from the stress of following rules? | 33 |
| 2.26 | Is there a benefit similar to meditation from doing the form slow? | 33 |
| 2.27 | If tai chi is a martial art, why do the form slowly? How does that prepare a person to fight? Fights, after all, happen fast. | 34 |

## III. TAI CHI & SELF-DEFENSE

| | | |
|---|---|---|
| 3.1 | Is tai chi just for good health? | 35 |
| 3.2 | Do we get the same benefits learning tai chi for health as we do when learning it for self-defense? | 35 |
| 3.3 | Am I missing something if I don't learn tai chi as self-defense? | 36 |
| 3.4 | But what if I am not interested in learning self-defense? | 36 |
| 3.5 | Why should one engage in a practice aimed at hurting others? | 37 |
| 3.6 | What makes tai chi unique and effective as a system of self-defense? | 38 |
| 3.7 | What is "yielding" in tai chi? | 38 |
| 3.8 | What is internal power? | 39 |
| 3.9 | You mentioned rootedness in self-defense. What exactly is it? | 39 |

| | |
|---|---:|
| 3.10 What is full-body integration? | 39 |
| 3.11 Is too much yielding bad or unbalanced? | 40 |
| 3.12 Tai Chi has an image that is very different from what most people associate with "martial arts." | 40 |
| 3.13 Other martial arts seem easier and faster to learn. | 41 |
| 3.14 What makes martial art fighting different from a bar fight? | 41 |
| 3.15 If tai chi is a fighting art, why are some of its movements so flowing and aesthetically pleasing to the eye? Combat, more often than not, is brutal and chaotic. Explain the paradox. | 42 |
| 3.16 People have such different types of energy. While yielding, I feel like I am losing myself —I become a chameleon, adapting to each person. How do I yield but also maintain my own goal and energy? | 42 |
| 3.17 How can we learn how to fight if we practice in "slow-motion"? | 43 |
| 3.18 Is it true that no matter how slow our pace is, we should always work at going slower? | 43 |
| 3.19 Does tai chi develop confidence in fighting? | 44 |
| 3.20 Is tai chi self-defense suitable for women? | 44 |
| 3.21 In addition to using the attributes of tai chi to overcome a stronger opponent, can they be used against more than one opponent? | 45 |
| 3.22 Is tai chi fighting something I can pick up quickly? | 45 |
| 3.23 How many years of practice are required before one can successfully apply tai chi fighting techniques in the outside world? | 46 |
| 3.24. Why is the palm used more than the fist in tai chi? | 46 |
| 3.25 How do you make your palm stronger, how do you train your fist? | 46 |
| 3.26 How does a relaxed fist that is trained correctly penetrate deeper than a stiff one? | 47 |
| 3.27 What are Silk Reeling and Spiral Power? Are The Compass, Rhino Gazes at the Moon, Owl Turns His Head and Cloud Hands (Stationary feet) examples of Silk-Reeling exercises? | 48 |
| 3.28 In fighting, do we ever set a trap to lure an opponent? | 48 |
| 3.29 When striking an opponent, what is the correct distance to place oneself for maximum power? | 49 |
| 3.30 Have you ever had to use self-defense in real life? | 49 |

## IV. LEARNING TAI CHI

| | |
|---|---:|
| 4.1 Is tai chi for everyone? | 50 |
| 4.2 Can I learn tai chi from books or videos? | 50 |
| 4.3 What is the correct way of learning the form? | 51 |
| 4.4 Please explain the process of teaching tai chi one move at a time. | 51 |
| 4.5 Do these smaller parts become one move later on? | 52 |
| 4.6 Why am I told to make a ball with my hands as I first learn the form? | 52 |
| 4.7 What do you mean by 'approximation'? How many approximations are there? | 53 |
| 4.8 Why am I leaning forward to tuck in? How does this help my alignment and *chi* flow? | 53 |
| 4.9 When being round, can I just point my shoulders in — why must I concave my chest? | 54 |
| 4.10 How can I suspend my head while leaning forward, concave my chest, and do the move — isn't this too much to do at the same time? | 55 |
| 4.11 In simple terms, please list the basic tai chi principles a beginner should keep in mind. | 55 |
| 4.12 You mention alignment all the time. Why is alignment so important in tai chi? | 56 |

4.13 What are corrections? Why do people who have been doing tai chi for a long time and even teaching tai chi still come to class for corrections? 56
4.14 Do corrections ever end? 57
4.15 What, specifically, is the best path to progress? 58
4.16 How do you learn the most from a teacher? 59
4.17 Can you give another example of following curriculum? 60
4.18 Do some students take a long time to learn the form? 60
4.19 Do some students learn the form faster than others? 61
4.20 So what would be an ideal student? 61
4.21 Why is it so important to be a good student? 62
4.22 What's the best way to motivate myself to reach a higher-level in tai chi and *nei kung*? 62
4.23 How does one judge his progress in tai chi, *nei kung* and meditation? 62
4.24 After the Short Form, are there other forms to learn? 63
4.25 Why breathe in when striking, both in the form and when fighting? 64

# V. PRACTICING TAI CHI

5.1 It seems that tai chi does not emphasize discipline to the degree that other systems do. 66
5.2 Should there be any pain when practicing tai chi? 66
5.3 Why lean forward and round the back? I thought the back should be straight and vertical in Tai Chi? 67
5.4 Are there other reasons why we should lean forward? 68
5.5 Do we also lean back? 68
5.6 What is the importance of smoothness in practicing tai chi? 68
5.7 We learn the tai chi form very meticulously. How do we bridge the gap between including all the details of the form and achieving smoothness? 69
5.8 How do you coordinate breathing to slow movement in tai chi? 69
5.9 Can the slow movement of tai chi benefit the cardiovascular system? 69
5.10 In what way does slow movement benefit the cardiovascular system? 70
5.11 What is continuous form? 70
5.12 What should our state of mind be while doing the tai chi form? Are we visualizing the *chi* flow? 71
5.13 There is more to practicing the fast form than just doing the form faster. What else should we concentrate on? 72
5.14 Is it ever a good idea to break up the form to work on specific moves or sections? 72
5.15 Is the tai chi form continuous from beginning to end without stopping? 72
5.16 Should the tai chi form be done at the same height? 73
5.17 Will doing the form slowly and correctly over a long period of time give me great internal power and speed? 73
5.18 Why is the *qua* so important? 74
5.19 Why are some postures done only on one side? Is this unbalanced? 74
5.20 Does it become boring to practice the same form every day for the rest of your life? Isn't there something else to learn? 75
5.21 If tai chi is a complete martial art, why should I also practice meditation, *chi kung* and *nei kung*? 76

| | | |
|---|---|---|
| 5.22 | I've completed the short form and a correction. What should I do next? | 76 |
| 5.23 | How does Push-Hands training strengthen the Tai Chi Form? | 76 |
| 5.24 | I've read several books on push-hands and they all discuss it as a competition between two people to see who can maintain their root and balance. Why don't we ever play this game in class? What is the point of push-hands? | 77 |
| 5.25 | What are some of the main differences between the way people train today and the way they trained in the past? | 78 |
| 5.26 | Some practitioners of hard style kung fu wear weighted hand bands or wrist weights to increase their strength. Should we do this while practicing tai chi? | 79 |
| 5.27 | What's the best way to train? | 79 |
| 5.28 | What is the ultimate goal of practicing? | 80 |
| 5.29 | How can a person undertake to do tai chi "perfectly"? | 80 |
| 5.30 | How can we overcome the inertia of not practicing tai chi, when we know tai chi is good for us? | 80 |
| 5.31 | How can we make practice a priority? | 81 |
| 5.32 | How does negative thinking keep us from practicing? | 81 |
| 5.33 | How do we cultivate a positive mindset? | 81 |
| 5.34 | If we only have 45 minutes to an hour per day to dedicate to *nei kung*, tai chi and *Eternal Spring*, should we split our time among those practices? | 82 |
| 5.35 | What if we have physical pain and don't feel like practicing? | 82 |
| 5.36 | In what order should I practice meditation, *nei kung* and tai chi? | 82 |
| 5.37 | I live far from the city and can only come to tai chi class for corrections occasionally. What is the best way to enhance my practice? | 83 |
| 5.38 | After taking two or three classes consecutively in the evening, sleep is difficult. Do you recommend any sort of "cool down" breathing techniques or other exercises to help ease the body into sleep? | 83 |

## VI. TAI CHI, *CHI KUNG* & *NEI KUNG*

| | | |
|---|---|---|
| 6.1 | What is *chi kung*? | 84 |
| 6.2 | What is *nei kung*? | 84 |
| 6.3 | Please explain the difference between *chi kung* and *nei kung*. | 85 |
| 6.4 | If *nei kung* is a more intense level of developing *chi*, why bother with *chi kung* at all? | 85 |
| 6.5 | Can the development of *chi* be felt during *nei kung* and *chi kung*? | 86 |
| 6.6 | Other teachers say the toes should be turned out during *chi kung* exercises generally but also during Horse Stance specifically, but you say 'toes in.' Why is this? | 87 |
| 6.7 | Is it important to follow the order of the exercises in the *Eternal Spring* and *Nei Kung* books? | 88 |
| 6.8 | What is the concept behind the order of the *Eternal Spring* series? | 88 |
| 6.9 | What is the concept behind the order of the *Nei Kung* series? | 89 |
| 6.10 | In between *Eternal Spring Chi Kung* exercises we open our mouths and breathe out audibly. Why do we do this? | 90 |
| 6.11 | What is the purpose of Roaring Lion in *Eternal Spring*? | 91 |
| 6.12 | When we start the Horse Stance, at what height should we be? Should we start low, medium, or high? Why? | 91 |

| | | |
|---|---|---|
| 6.13 | Please explain in more detail the three stages of developing the back in Embracing Horse. | 92 |
| 6.14 | What should "lasting forever" feel like? | 92 |
| 6.15 | If you are in correct alignment, should your legs be feeling relaxed or is it normal to experience some degree of muscle strain? | 92 |
| 6.16 | During Horse Stance, should I be "doing" anything? | 93 |
| 6.17 | How can *nei kung* help develop muscle strength in the upper body? Can it substitute for weight training? | 93 |
| 6.18 | Does high-level *chi kung* and *nei kung* training strengthen the body's weakest points like the eyes, kidneys and groin? | 94 |
| 6.19 | What does one need to watch out for if one is practicing too much *nei kung*? | 95 |
| 6.20 | How do *chi kung*, *nei kung*, and tai chi exercise the organs? | 95 |
| 6.21 | Is *nei kung* some kind of bulletproof vest? | 95 |
| 6.22 | What is the chief benefit or pay-off for doing *nei kung*? | 96 |
| 6.23 | Does *nei kung* strengthen the knees? | 96 |
| 6.24 | What additional *nei kung* exercises are there? | 97 |
| 6.26 | Are there psychological benefits of doing *nei kung*? | 97 |

## VII. TAI CHI AND MEDITATION

| | | |
|---|---|---|
| 7.1 | There are so many different kinds of meditation systems, each with its own philosophy. How do they compare with what you teach? | 99 |
| 7.2 | What is Taoist meditation? | 99 |
| 7.3 | Is it easy to discover your individual Tao? | 100 |
| 7.4 | Is meditation an important part of tai chi training? | 100 |
| 7.5 | What does meditation have to do with self-defense? | 101 |
| 7.6 | What's the difference between the standing meditation of Horse Stance and the lotus position of sitting meditation? | 101 |
| 7.7 | Why is "quiet sitting" good for us? | 101 |
| 7.8 | How does having a strong mind help us in our daily life? | 102 |
| 7.9 | What other benefits can be gained from this type of meditation? | 102 |
| 7.10 | Can you further elaborate on the benefits of Taoist meditation practice? | 103 |
| 7.11 | In class, you mentioned that we develop "subconscious awareness" by practicing quiet sitting. What do you mean by this? | 103 |
| 7.12 | How does one move the *chi* within the body: with the mind or will? Is this a dangerous practice? | 104 |
| 7.13 | How can quietness be achieved in the city where it is noisy and hectic? | 104 |
| 7.14 | Meditation seems easy. A person is just sitting there doing nothing. Should we learn meditation first, before learning *Eternal Spring*, tai chi or *nei kung*? | 105 |
| 7.15 | Does thinking use up a lot of energy? | 106 |
| 7.16 | What does it mean to short-circuit the system? | 106 |
| 7.17 | Does positive thinking drain the body? | 106 |
| 7.18 | How long does it take before someone experiences *chi* during meditation? | 106 |
| 7.19 | Can you describe some examples of feeling *chi*? | 107 |
| 7.20 | Do you feel *chi* along the meridians? | 107 |
| 7.21 | While meditating, is it correct to visualize the *chi* going through the body? | 107 |

| | |
|---|---:|
| 7.22 Should we try to move the *chi* throughout the body? | 107 |
| 7.23 Besides improving *chi*, what are the benefits of meditation? | 108 |
| 7.24 Is there any other step I can take to achieve quietness (*jing*)? | 108 |
| 7.25 Why does emptying the mind feel terrifying, like a little "death"? | 109 |

## VIII. TAI CHI AND SEX

| | |
|---|---:|
| 8.1 What is the Taoist view on sex? | 111 |
| 8.2 How does tai chi affect sex? | 111 |
| 8.3 What do fighting arts have to do with sex? | 112 |
| 8.4 Is sex good for health? | 113 |
| 8.5 Can sex without release increase the body's *chi*? | 113 |
| 8.6 I thought Taoist monks practice celibacy. | 114 |
| 8.7 Why are religions so obsessed with sex? | 114 |
| 8.8 What is your opinion about sex in a civilized society? | 114 |
| 8.9 What would make us civilized with regard to sex? | 115 |
| 8.10 What does marriage have to do with sex? | 115 |
| 8.11 Do you support sex education in schools? | 116 |
| 8.12 What happens when we suppress sexual energy? | 116 |
| 8.13 What about people who consider sex obscene? | 117 |
| 8.14 What about violence and sex? | 117 |
| 8.15 How can the average person benefit from your teaching regarding sex? | 118 |

## IX. TAI CHI IN DAILY LIFE

| | |
|---|---:|
| 9.1 What impact can tai chi have on daily life? | 119 |
| 9.2 Can this yielding apply to any situation? | 119 |
| 9.3 How do I yield my way into a better job? | 120 |
| 9.4 What if I look for a long time and still can't get a job I want? | 120 |
| 9.5 If I practice tai chi, will I really see progress in other areas of my life? | 121 |
| 9.6 What can I study to round out a quality tai chi lifestyle? | 121 |
| 9.7 Do you think that tai chi and meditation can resolve world issues? | 122 |
| 9.8 Can you give specific examples of the type of "organized powers" that stand in the way of a more humane and more reasoned society? | 122 |
| 9.9 I understand that you plan on explaining how Taoism can help in a future book, could you just briefly explain how these powers stymie social progress? | 123 |
| 9.10 So what would a more humane world look like? | 124 |
| 9.11 In what way does tai chi encompass a spiritual component? | 125 |

| | |
|---|---:|
| Afterword: The Tao, The World, and Beyond | 126 |
| *Wu Wei* — 'Let it be.' | 126 |
| It's Not Easy Though — So How Can This Be Achieved? | 127 |
| Tai Chi is a Counterweight to Nihilism | 127 |
| Just Do It | 129 |
| Glossary | 131 |

# NOTE ON THIS TEXT

This text is a sequel to *Tai Chi Chuan Principles & Practice* (*TCCP&P*). The spellings and italicizations used in the publications of CK Chu Tai Chi were set during the publication process of *TCCP&P* decades ago. Our language, therefore, varies from the *pinyin* format that is becoming the standard Romanization of Chinese terms. Thus, this text, for example, uses *"chi"* where many texts are using *"qi"*. Throughout this text, Chinese words are italicized, like *chi*, unless they have been adopted into English, like kung fu and tai chi. Unlike *TCCP&P*, this text does not contain the Chinese characters for words common to tai chi discourse. The reader seeking those characters should consult *TCCP&P*.

# FOREWORD:
## *The Story of CK and Chu Tai Chi*

I was born in Hong Kong in 1937. There, as in China, kung fu was a normal part of life just like, in America, baseball and football are a normal part of life. In fact, in my elementary school Master See taught Northern Shaolin style as part of gym class. At the age of 12, I began more serious kung fu training by studying Fut Ga (Buddha Fist), which is a relatively obscure style from Southern China. Later I added judo and both Wu and Yang style tai chi to my studies. Knowing kung fu, in other words, was not unusual but I never thought I'd open my own tai chi school.

I came to this country to study Physics and, until 1995, taught physics, first in college and then in high school. While in graduate school, I had stopped my martial arts training and by the end I didn't like the feeling of being out of shape. Since you cannot practice martial arts without partners, once out of graduate school I resumed my practice of martial arts at William CC Chen's school, really the only tai chi school at that time. I also resumed judo practice at the Judo Center in the East 70's.

From my own research and practice I had come to understand that tai chi is the best system of health and self-defense yet devised but it is also the most difficult and, for that reason, most misunderstood. Recognizing that the best way for me to continue my practice was to teach tai chi, I taught the Yang style tai chi form as a class at Aaron Bank's Karate Academy in Manhattan and Hank Kraft's Judo School in Queens after my regular work hours. I had so many students I decided to open my own school to accommodate them all.

Unlike today, when you can find yoga, tai chi, and martial arts schools in many areas of the city, the few schools back then were located mostly in Chinatown. I wanted to take tai chi to the world so I opened the Tai Chi Chuan Center in 1973 in the Times Square neighborhood, crossroads of the country. Bryant Park was a bit shabby then and Times Square, in those days, was not bright and shiny — nor was it full of tourists. The city was bankrupt and the heart of the city was seedy but interesting: my car was stolen; an annoying bum who would ask for change all the time outside the school turned out to be an undercover cop; students reported having to use their tai chi to defend themselves in the subway. My school, opening in the days of Bruce Lee's fame, was part of a newfound interest in kung fu among Americans and I had a lot of students. The first school was small and classes would be really crowded. Most students who came to my school then, and nearly all who have come since, want to study tai chi to improve their health, but a handful have come wanting to study tai chi to fight.

Martial arts were new in the United States then and, with some difficulty, the nascent martial arts community staged tournaments where students could test their skills and schools compete with one another. Tournaments were a good opportunity to see whether a school was authentic, that is, whether its training curriculum produced good fighters or not. A handful of my students wanted to participate in these tournaments so I agreed to train them. To make sure they were strong enough to take punishment from an opponent's strikes and kicks, I taught them my *nei kung* system and my meditation technique. Now, *nei kung* was, and in many ways still is, one of those secrets written and discussed a great deal but few people really understand it. In fact, just about everyone in China has heard of *nei kung* as some kind of inner power that makes fighters invulnerable to an opponent's strikes but precious few know what it entails. Not surprisingly, there are many myths and legends about *nei kung* — much of it silly nonsense. People perform an incredible feat of strength or endurance and call it *nei kung* (there are many examples now online). Most such tales and claims are bogus. *Nei Kung* is a set of exercises used as an adjunct to form training that increases the overall health and integrity of the whole body. The result is increased strength, endurance, and internal power so that the body becomes so strong it is practically immune to being struck and kicked. The body is also capable of delivering very powerful strikes. The effectiveness of tai chi and *nei kung* cannot be realized unless accompanied by a solid and consistent meditation practice. The mind has to be trained to work with the body.

From the mid-1970s to early 1980s, in tournaments in Boston and New York, my students demonstrated the effectiveness and power of tai chi by winning many titles. In general, there remains a fundamental misunderstanding of tai chi: most people think of tai chi as a slow series of movement done by the infirm and, thus, incapable of making a fighter powerful. Opponents often exclaimed, "how can *they* beat us?" They have no understanding of tai chi and did not know of Yang Wu Di, Invincible Yang, or the feats of skill of past tai chi masters. People didn't mind losing, so long as it wasn't to some tai chi sissy. This bias even affected judges as many times we thought we won but the judges voted for their own fighter, from their school. Because of tournament politics, it was best to win with a knockout. I remember my student, Steve James, fighting to the booing of the crowd at a tournament in Chinatown. Steve was *yielding* to his opponent quite well to my eye but in the eye of the crowd, Steve was a coward. They could not see that he was looking for the right position. As they were shaking their heads at what they perceived as the weakness of tai chi, the opponent suddenly fell to the ground. Just about everyone, including the referee who had forgotten to start the knock-out count, was shocked. "What had happened?" "How could this be?" were the questions being asked around the room. Through the shock I yelled for the ref to start counting: he did. Steve won by yielding and then delivering a fast, but powerful straight punch that laid the opponent out. He illustrated the basic tai chi principle: yield to master the situation and then strike.

While spectators remained ignorant of tai chi, my students won the respect — a grudging, surprised respect — of opposing schools, a respect which reverberates to this day. Some thirty years later, opponents from back then have told me how afraid they were of my students because their most powerful strike or kick wouldn't make my students flinch. That is the internal power derived from *nei kung* training. I still remember how Edmund Berry could allow a full blow to touch any part of his body, including his face, and roll with it. This is the level of skill one gains through practicing push-hands. To the opponent who delivers what he thinks is a dead-on knockout punch, it can be quite deflating to see his best punch prove ineffective. The fight really ends there for the opponent; of course tournaments don't work that way. On the other hand, tai chi fighters have a power in their strike that is so subtle and penetrating it may not be felt immediately. I remember Vincent Sobers' championship fight at Madison Square Gardens when the referee became impatient because the opponent did not come to the center to resume fighting when called. The opponent could not move because of the punch to the abdomen he had received from Sobers in the previous round. Culminating this period of New York tournaments was the largest martial arts tournament at Madison Square Gardens in 1981. Vincent Sobers, in the middleweight division, and Richard Trybulski, in the heavyweight division, both won titles by knockout. Unfortunately, that tournament was the last great martial arts tournament in the city because of the difficulties of running a tournament in New York City.

Success in the tournaments bred imitation and copycats. Just like in the movies where people believe success is based on a secret move, not hard work and training, there were those who tried to discover our secret by filming us. This spying effort didn't help them though. I can show anyone how to do a Heel Kick, but to make it an effective weapon for fighting, you have to practice it thousands of times — and even then it cannot be removed from the whole tai chi training system. Kung fu in general is done fast, but some people tried just doing their movements or tai chi movements slow, because they saw us moving slow and thought that slowness was the key. But that is not enough either. Tai chi is based on the development of inner power through the training of proper alignment, breathing, integration and coordination of the body. You also need to study the tai chi form's applications, practice push-hands, and you must practice meditation. Tai chi is the most advanced martial art yet devised and there is nothing secret about it. Responding to the general misunderstanding of tai chi and to help my own students, I wrote *Tai Chi Chuan Principles & Practice* (1981). There, I simply showed that my curriculum is based on what the old masters say in the tai chi classics, not on some secret teaching I alone had received. This book, *Why Tai Chi?*, is in many ways a sequel to that first book. Here, I continue to explain why tai chi is superior to other systems as a fighting and healing art.

Originally, I taught *nei kung* to the half a dozen fighters in the school. I soon discovered they, in turn, were teaching *nei kung* to others within the school and I was faced with the problem of incorrect transmission. Being trained in an art is not the same as being able to train others. For this reason as well as the desire to use *nei kung* to help people who had no interest in fighting improve their health, I decided to hold workshops and teach a regular *Nei Kung* Class starting in the late 1970s. People came from other kung fu schools inside and outside New York to learn my *Nei Kung* system. Realizing my students needed and wanted a simple how-to book and knowing that no such book existed, with the help of my students Jim Borrelli and John Shramko, I put together the first ever how-to book on *nei kung*, *The Book of Nei Kung* (1986). Ultimately, I certified Jim as an instructor. He was the first person to be certified in my system. He opened a school in Los Angeles.

Of course, not everyone who came to the school came to fight and we were not fighting all the time. Most people come to my school in Times Square to improve or recover their health. Then, as now, the school was a community of people seeking to renew their own humanity and, by extension, renew the world. Together, this community held and continues to hold an annual celebration of the Chinese New Year. These banquets have always been a time for bonding as well as demonstrations of the tai chi form, weapons, push-hands, and applications. For twenty years, we went on an annual weekend retreat at Ananda Ashram at Monroe, New York. There, we enjoyed the outdoors while continuing tai chi studies with classes in meditation, tai chi, *nei kung*, and push-hands as well as discussions on Taoist philosophy and life. Whenever the opportunity has arisen, we have also sought to promote tai chi to the general public with appearances on TV, the Fifth Avenue Book Fair, and demonstrations in Chinatown, at school clubs, and World Tai Chi Day in Bryant Park.

In the mid-1990s, new tournaments were begun in the New York area and Hugh Marlowe wanted to make his bid for a title. I had my doubts about his prospects, but it turned out that fighting classes at my school were tougher than the fights at this tournament — he was more than ready. This tournament featured the *lei tai* stage, which is a raised platform without ropes. I have a vivid memory of one of his fights: Hugh knocked his opponent off the platform. The opponent landed on the floor and started convulsing. Nobody seemed to know what to do to help him, so I rushed over and revived him. Everyone was so surprised and shocked by what had happened, nobody bothered to thank me for reviving him. Once again, people were surprised and dismayed by the power of tai chi. Marlowe won the heavyweight division of the 1995 New York Chinese Martial Art Championship and Tri-State Kung Fu Full Contact tournament by knock-outs: two tournaments in a row, on the same weekend.

Tai chi is the best exercise ever devised and anyone can do it with the proper instruction and approach to training. With such a beginning, possible only by learning the art from a master, anyone can reap the benefits of this art. Yet there is no getting around the fact that the beginning period of tai chi training can be taxing to the body, especially for those people who are in poor shape. I had long been asking myself: how could I help people who are not fit enough to do tai chi but would greatly benefit from it? Upon retiring from high school teaching in 1995, I devoted myself to answering this question by devising a *chi kung* system that would prepare anyone for the rigors of tai chi practice. I called it *Eternal Spring Chi Kung* and it turned out to be good for everybody, no matter what their level, because it is really a drill in such basic things as breathing that is necessary to everyone's training and life — we must breathe to live, so why not breathe better!

Readers appreciated the simple, straightforward manner of *The Book of Nei Kung* so I used the how-to approach in two more books, *Chu Meditation* (2002) and *Eternal Spring Chi Kung* (2003). *Chu Meditation* was a long time coming since I started teaching meditation so that *nei kung* practitioners could calm their mind during exercise and reap the benefits. But meditation practice is vital in this world of over-stressed people and I hope the book helps some people relax. The how-to format left out an explanation of Taoist philosophy so the reader could get right to it. A forthcoming book, however, will detail the nine steps of Taoist self-cultivation. Again, with the help of Jim Borrelli, the *Eternal Spring* book simply instructs the reader how to do *chi kung*. Thus, my school now had a complete curriculum of internal system training with four core disciplines (meditation, *chi kung*, *nei kung*, and tai chi for health and self-defense) as well as the advanced studies of push-hands, fighting, and weapons.

To further my conviction that tai chi is a solution to health problems as well as the best self-defense system, we established a separate, public service entity called the Tai Chi Chuan Center Inc. as a non-profit organization in 2000. The school continued its mission to teach my curriculum under the name Chu Tai Chi (it became CK Chu Tai Chi in 2010). For the last 10 years, the Tai Chi Chuan Center has facilitated the teaching of *Eternal Spring* in senior centers, churches, and parks. In 2003, the Tai Chi Chuan Center began its most successful outreach program to date. Starting in May, volunteer students teach an early morning combined *Eternal Spring Chi Kung*/Tai Chi class in Bryant Park for free throughout the summer. Through this program we have greatly improved the public's understanding of tai chi and enabled more than a few people to learn the art when, due to time or money constraints, they might not have.

Tournament fever returned to the school from 2004-2006, when a contingent of students went to the United States Kuo Shu Federation (USKSF) Championship Tournament in Baltimore. Since its inception in the 1990s, the USKSF has become one of the toughest, best run tournaments in the United States. Mostly, participants in these tournaments are in their twenties. However, Hyland Harris proved the value of tai chi training by competing one year at the age of 38 — he knocked out a guy half his age and earned a medal. Another student participated in the tournament for three years in a row. In his first fight, John Signoriello knocked his opponent down almost instantly and the medics had to take the opponent away. We could hear someone in the audience moan, "not to a tai chi guy." One time, John used a Heel Kick to his opponent's head, knocking him off the *lei tai* platform to win a fight. The spectators went wild; they couldn't believe tai chi was so powerful. John was undefeated for two years in the Middleweight B Division. John then joined the US team to fight in Singapore in 2006 and the USKSF later voted him competitor of the year.

Today, CK Chu Tai Chi teaches four basic disciplines as well as advanced training. We also have a teacher certification program for those who wish to further their understanding of tai chi and who want to advance the development of the art of tai chi in the future. This certification program is modeled on the university system with transparent requirements that advance the art and science of tai chi, not any lineage. My curriculum is taught in Italy, Venezuela, and Los Angeles. Recently, I consulted on the creation of the Martial Arts Studies B.A. Program at the University of Bridgeport in Connecticut. This program is the only one of its kind in the U.S. and my student, Dan Zegibe, teaches my system as part of the curriculum, using my books as the official textbooks for the course.

Tai chi remains the most difficult and the most misunderstood art in the world; students and teachers wonder why this, why that, why do the form slowly, why align the body this way and not that… This book will hopefully answer those questions and help clear the misunderstandings of tai chi so people will aim for the correct path. It is important that everybody recognize there are no secrets or need to depend on lineage claims. Rather, a properly taught tai chi curriculum can be pursued by anyone at any age and in any shape or health condition. To further the spread of tai chi and, with it, improved health, I offer this text. I hope you are able to read the book many times as you will get a deeper and deeper understanding as you read and practice the art. The more understanding you have on the subject, the more enjoyment you have. It is my hope that this book will inspire more people to do tai chi.

Keep practicing.

— C. K. Chu
June 2010

# INTRODUCTION
## *Tai Chi is a Fighting Art*

Tai Chi Chuan or tai chi is the most widely practiced exercise in the world and yet very few people know its true nature. Since opening my tai chi school, CK Chu Tai Chi, in Times Square in 1973, I have taught several thousand people — some for a short time and some for a long time — and I am still amazed at how tai chi is misconceived in the West. People think it is a New Age dance or ritual to be performed on occasion. That's incorrect. Tai chi is kung fu; it is an internal system of martial art, a very sophisticated art of self-defense. But tai chi is not just another skill or another technique for overcoming an opponent. Rather, it is a way of life, a way of being human. Tai chi encompasses Taoism's desire to develop human nature fully through a training regimen that maximizes the body's health and longevity. Tai chi, in that sense, is Taoism expressed. Practicing tai chi means expressing the full beauty of the body and mind while maintaining a constructive and realistic way to approach life in all its dimensions.

Although tai chi is an art of defense, that does not mean it is not also an art of offense. When executed correctly, self-defense is a prerequisite to an accurate, timely offense. Generally, people associate fighting with violence and aggression and they do not want to be a part of it. But there are always those who want to commit violence on others. Therefore, the purpose of self-defense training is to be able to handle a situation in which a confrontation turns violent. It is part of the nature of any animal to be able to defend itself. Humans are no different. A cat, for example, falls onto its back as a round ball so as best to utilize its claws but elks step back for an antler-first charge. Humans also have a means of self-defense and likewise utilize the body to its maximum potential. However, whereas animals defend themselves instinctively, humans have lost this instinct as part of the civilizing process — we defer to authority figures like parents, teachers, and cops and let them defend us. With tai chi, we can return to defending ourselves rather than hoping others can do it for us.

Learning how to utilize self-defense techniques inevitably trains the body and mind. Tai chi training does not to make you aggressive but makes you able to overcome aggression aimed at you. "Fighting," in other words, is the natural way to train the body most effectively. By following tai chi principles, the whole body and mind become healthy and strong. You may never have to fight in your whole life but you know you can handle it should it arise. Plus, the health benefits enable you to live your life to its fullest.

To be able to achieve the full benefits of tai chi, a student must go through a certain kind of training: learning to do the form slowly, working on coordination, balance, and the body's conditioning; executing the form fast and application of the form's movements to real fighting situations. Learning tai chi step by step is excellent for health. Many people do the beginning part of tai chi training and reap its health benefits. A few go further. Whichever category you are in, you may be confident that the value of tai chi is inexhaustible and you will get out of it what you put into it.

## Tai Chi is Science, Art, and Philosophy

Tai chi is a science, art, and philosophy in one. There is an ultimate way to move the body with a mind connection and it is not subjective. Tai chi has a structure. It has its own kinds of laws and elements — these make the tai chi system unique. There are basic principles that, like laws, must be observed at all times. The laws were set down in writing by the old masters. I included my translations of these classics in my first book, *Tai Chi Chuan Principles & Practice*. In the classics, the old masters' love of tai chi is obvious, and they explained the principles of the science of tai chi eloquently. Like any science, tai chi is always moving forward. We are standing on the old masters' shoulders while exploring further.

Within the tai chi structure, however, there is ample room for flexibility, creativity, and individual exploration. Execution of the tai chi form in observance of the principles is an expression of the beauty of the human form in movement — having poise, balance, coordination, and power. In executing tai chi as a solo exercise, the self is fully expressed. The old masters spoke of the 'tai chi feeling' attained after repeating the form many times consecutively. The feeling is similar to climbing a high mountain — the higher you go, the clearer you see. You feel as calm as the empty sky and fluid as the river. It is a feeling of ecstasy as you experience the oneness of your mind and body and your oneness with nature.

However, although tai chi is often thought of as a solo performance, it is actually the study of responding to another human. Tai chi is the art of responding and the same principles used to respond to a fighting situation can be applied to everyday life. As in dance (and dance and fighting are related in many ways), there is beauty in the elegance of response to another. Therefore, tai chi is an art — the art of fighting. Responding to a violent act beautifully is an art — the art of resolving problems. Suppose you are attacked but you gracefully, artfully step aside and the attacker flies past. Nobody gets hurt and the attacker knows he is beaten. There is no need for further violence. Tai chi is that art. The beauty of tai chi is that, by following its principles your body will move naturally and you will come to realize that any other way of moving is clumsy and unnatural. The more you do tai chi, the greater your experience of the beauty of the art of fighting. It all depends on understanding the science as well as the philosophy of tai chi.

Tai chi philosophy is based on the basic principle of *yin* and *yang*: in any dynamic situation there exists both action and reaction. Through an understanding of this simple notion of complementarity, you will know how to respond to and resolve situations occurring in life. In tai chi, the application of this principle is summed up using one beautiful phrase: "I utilize four ounces to deflect a thousand pounds" (*Tai Chi Chuan Principles & Practice*, *TCCP&P*, p. 102). This means you should use just enough energy to deflect the force of the adverse situation rather than trying to muster an equal overpowering and opposite force. Very likely you cannot match the incoming force and if you try, you will be destroyed. Better to know how to deflect it. This philosophy is very useful in fighting where you need to be able to respond to any attack appropriately. The art of tai chi includes learning mind and body coordination and integration. Tai chi is the art of fighting, of health and of life. It is also the art of the virtuous human being. Based on Taoism, tai chi teaches you how to be calm, centered, flexible, pliable, and, like a child, curious about yourself and the world. Further, it teaches you to enjoy life, enjoy yourself, and enjoy others.

## Western Exercise

Most Western exercises are done to gain superficial looks, muscular development, endurance for marathons, and bodybuilding contests. To me, this is off the mark. The so-called Mr. Universe body is not the way the human body should look and move. Can you imagine an animal with the overdeveloped muscles of Mr. Universe? The animal would move very inefficiently and without beauty. We tend to glorify competition and extreme body exercises like a marathon. Running over 26 miles abuses the body. Even horses do not run 26 miles all the time. We are human and have our own characteristics and uniqueness. We need a way to efficiently develop and move the body and respond to any situation. Tai chi is that way.

For example, muscle building and running are one-dimensional exercises — doing them you accomplish one thing, while adding mileage to the body. Tai chi is the correct way to develop the entire body while taking off the mileage accumulated in daily life. Plus, you can continue to practice it throughout your entire life. This is in contrast to the Olympic gymnasts that people find fascinating. He or she can be champion at 16, but will have to retire before the age of 21. A correct exercise like tai chi can be practiced at any age, even when you're 90 years old and beyond.

# THIS BOOK

Over the years students have asked me many questions of "why tai chi this?" and "why tai chi that?" and "why does tai chi work?" I've been accumulating these questions and have decided to answer the most essential and common ones in this book to show the full spectrum of tai chi. My hope is that, by reading the questions and answers, people will gain insight into what tai chi really is. I've put the questions in different categories to show the full range of what tai chi encompasses — health, self-defense, meditation, sex, and daily life.

This book is designed for both beginning and advanced students. Beginners who read it may be inspired to learn more about tai chi. Advanced students will get a comprehensive idea of tai chi and what the possibilities are for them. Of course, every level of student can benefit from the "nitty-gritty" of what is *chi*, root, push-hands, *yin* and *yang* and other topics. The book can be read from beginning to end or picked up in any section or topic and reread many times. It's written in the style of light reading, but the questions and answers are very solid.

As I said, tai chi is an art form and, like any art, the more you understand the better your craft will be. It is not just some physical exercise like running on a treadmill or doing push-ups or sit-ups. Rather, like other disciplines, the more you do it and the more you understand, the better your tai chi and the more there is to do and to learn. A tai chi practitioner is like a musician: the more he pursues his music, the better his music will be. If he is satisfied by just playing a few songs, then his craft will never improve. The same with tai chi.

You benefit from tai chi even on the first day you start learning. However, the more you practice the more you will know about tai chi, the more you will benefit and tai chi will become more compelling. Like science's endless pursuit of knowledge, studying tai chi leads deeper and deeper into an unknown universe. A beginner will focus on the principles of tai chi. Later on, an advanced student will encompass all aspects of tai chi in body and mind and coordination, becoming more grounded, rounded and relaxed.

Tai Chi has been capturing people's minds and bodies for close to a thousand years. There have also been many studies of the benefits of tai chi. Doing even a little tai chi correctly will put you far ahead of where you would be doing many other exercises. This book will tell you how to train and the benefits will be ten or a hundred fold. It is my hope people will understand tai chi and make it part of their life.

Because some terminology may be confusing, I have included a glossary as a reference. No matter how ambitious I am in answering questions, there is always one more question to be answered. The idea of this book is to provide enough Q&A's to help your practice of tai chi. I have planted the seed and hopefully the seed will grow for a hundred or a thousand years, like a redwood tree. I believe there are enough ingredients in the book to allow you to move forward to as high a level as you want to attain.

# I. WHAT IS TAI CHI?

## 1.1
### What is tai chi chuan?

Tai Chi Chuan (or *taijiquan* in *pinyin*), commonly known as "tai chi," is a sophisticated and ancient Chinese martial arts system comprised of movements that have both self-defense applications and health benefits. In order to be a good fighter, a person must have good health. By practicing Tai Chi Chuan, one will inevitably develop a strong and flexible body, and a focused, alert mind. A fighter must be strong, alert, and responsive. His or her body and mind must be integrated in order to be prepared for any situation. Regardless of the level of the practitioner, even if he only practices a small amount, he will receive large benefits. That is why Tai Chi Chuan is one of the most widely practiced martial arts in the world. (For more information on this question, see *Tai Chi Chuan Principles & Practice,* hereafter *TCCP&P,* p. 13).

## 1.2
### What is the origin of tai chi?

Chinese martial arts, commonly called Kung Fu or *wushu* are so old their invention is attributed to the mythical Yellow Emperor. Actually, the word for martial art, a developed fighting system, is *wushu* which means 'the art of combat.' Kung fu simply means having expertise or having acquired mastery in any set of skills, like cooking or carpentry. Early Chinese fighting systems were developed from careful observation of nature. Ancient fighters tried to learn from watching conflict between animals, seeking to understand why certain animals were strong or why apparently weaker animals won fights. Through such inquiry, techniques were created in imitation of animals. The results, called a *style*, often carried animal names, such as: White Crane Style, Tiger Style, or Praying Mantis Style. Later, with more study and experience, fighting styles became more organized and sometimes became institutionalized, often by temple monks.

Legend has it that a Taoist monk invented tai chi after having observed a long fight between a crane and a snake. Whatever the truth of this story, tai chi reflects the long tradition of Chinese *wushu* and is attributed to the Taoist monk Chang San-feng of the Southern Sung Dynasty (1127-1279 AD). Chang San-feng is believed to have synthesized tai chi into a coherent form and to have named it while residing at Wu-tang Mountain; sometimes tai chi is included with other styles developed in that area in the term 'Wu-tang system'. Of course, people practiced tai chi before him, but Chang is the one who is given the credit.

So while it is generally attributed to Chang San-feng, tai chi's origins are sketchy. As I mention in *Tai Chi Chuan Principles & Practice*:

> *"The origin is uncertain because in the martial arts, by the time the effectiveness of a new system is widely recognized, a few generations have gone by, thus creating a gap in history."*

### 1.3
### How does tai chi differ from other Chinese martial arts?

Chinese martial arts can be categorized into two traditions: external and internal. The external arts emphasize self-denial, martial discipline, and strengthening the body from the outside in. The most famous style of the external art is *Shaolin Chuan*, developed c. 575 C.E. at the Shaolin Temple — a Buddhist temple. So famous is this school that sometimes the external arts are simply called the Shaolin system. Students are disciplined by drillmasters who tell the students what to do and punish them if they fail. Training includes toughening exercises, like hitting the body (even the skull) or punching through boards to make the body insensitive to pain. Endurance exercises inure the body to pain. The fighting style uses a lot of jumping, hitting, emphasis on hand and foot, speed, calisthenics, and acrobatics. The goal of the external tradition is to overcome opponents with force — to use force against force, to be stronger, faster, tougher than the opponent.

Internal arts, the Wu-tang system mentioned above, include *hsing i, pa kua,* and tai chi. Internal arts strengthen the body from the inside out through *nei kung*, exercises that develop internal power (see Chapter 6). *Hsing i* is linear, emphasizing forceful straight-line attacks. *Pa kua* is a circular movement with specific movements concentrating on constant change of position *vis a vis* the opponent for both offensive and defensive advantage. These two arts complement each other so that, traditionally, people train to use them together. *Hsing i* is for attacking and *pa kua* for responding. *Hsing i* and *pa ku*a can be done through drills and by command. Tai chi, however, cannot be done unless you want to do it. Tai chi demands relaxation, which can only be developed through *nei kung* training and lots of solo practice. At my school, I emphasize *nei kung* training. This depends first and foremost on self-motivation and self-discipline. Nobody can command a person to do an internal art — the person has to want to do it for himself.

Tai chi is the *soft* style of the internal arts because there is no set strategy except yielding. Essentially, tai chi is the art of using 'four ounces against one thousand pounds.' External martial arts use force against force, and the other internal styles use repositioning. Tai chi uses the opponent's force against the opponent. In tai chi, the fighter stays in the center and through highly trained sensitivity responds to attacks from any direction. The training for this sensitivity is called Push-Hands. Through Push-Hands one learns yielding, the ability to sense the opponent's strength and energy, and the ability to respond to the opponent's attack. Tai chi is more sophisticated in theory and practice than any of the external arts; also, because it takes a long time for practitioners to develop the skills of this particular martial art, very few people understand it completely.

## 1.4
## What is the difference between tai chi and the other internal arts?

Tai chi comes from the application of the philosophy of Taoism to *wushu* and is the soft internal style. The Taoists wondered how a fighter on a battlefield or in a street fight could deal with any attack at any moment from any side. The answer to this was, in part, *jou* (pronounced 'yao,' see *TCCP&P* pp. 8, 65, 81, & 130). *Jou* is difficult to translate but more or less means 'soft' or 'flexible.' *Jou* is not weakness, but like a steel blade such as a double-edged sword — flexible but strong (and deadly). In tai chi, the goal is to bend to the opponent so as to counterattack where he is weakest. The idea can be seen in nature; an old tree's branches will break off in the wind but young trees and grasses bend to the wind. In tai chi, one aspires to be like the grass, not the rigid, brittle tree. Doing so depends on the tai chi artist staying calm and relaxed, able to deal with whatever comes —relaxed enough to respond with the body in whatever way the situation demands. All this is done while staying centered by responding with tai chi principles, like *yin* and *yang* (which means everything has a complement — if an attack is hard, I will be soft) and keeping the body round. Tai chi depends on understanding your self, the opponent, and the situation to know what is the best response for all concerned. Unlike the external styles, which simply seek to beat the opponent by overcoming him with a stronger attack, the tai chi artist can be weaker than the opponent and still win. This is possible because the tai chi artist lets the stronger attack come and exhaust itself and then counterattacks. Only the tai chi artist says, "I utilize only four ounces to deflect a thousand pounds" (from the "Song of Push-Hands," *TCCP&P* p. 102).

## 1.5
## What is Taoism?

Since the beginning of Chinese history, there has been discussion and pursuit of the reason behind things. It was discovered that there was a "law of the universe, or Tao" that was beyond any design (*TCCP&P*, p. 13). It was understood that humans could know reality, know nature, through observation and study. This study of the 'way of things' (or the 'way of nature') became the science called Taoism, which is a realistic and scientific approach to life that seeks to understand just what the 'way of things' is and then to go along with that way. The most famous book of Taoist insight is the *Tao Te Ching* by Lao Tzu. Over 2,500 years old, this book uses only 5,000 characters to express Tao philosophy. This tiny book not only influenced Chinese culture but the whole world. People around the world quote the *Tao Te Ching* without knowing it. For example, the saying, "a journey of a thousand miles begins beneath your feet" (or "with one step") is from the *Tao Te Ching* (chapter 64). Basically, Taoism is a science of humanity, a science of everything; the Tao of physics or health means there is a law of physics, like gravity, and there is a law of happiness and health.

## 1.6
## Is Taoism a religion?

Most people today think of Taoism as a religion because perhaps 90% of self-defined Taoists are religious or, at least, mystical in some way. This is a recent development. Originally, Taoism was the ceaseless asking and research into 'why things are the way they are.' But, in time, branches emerged that utilized religious or mystical methods in their inquiry into the Tao. Accordingly, various sects of religious Taoism have built temples and anointed priests to maintain the answers accumulated by this method. Similar to Christian denominations, these Taoist sects have competing views of the afterlife. They also have their immortals, people whose virtues made them so famous they are believed to have never died. The immortals are similar to angels or to saints in the West with some similarity to pagan, Greek or Hindu ideas of gods being present daily and everywhere.

## 1.7
## What kind of Taoist are you?

I adhere to the original scientific inquiry into the Tao, into why things are the way they are. That, to me, is Taoism. Further, I adhere to the traditional Taoist approach to health. Historically, Taoists have been realistic in their approach to health, knowing first and foremost that life is important as it is and should be enjoyed to the fullest. Thus, Taoists set about, systematically, to figure out the Tao of health. Applying this knowledge, Taoists hope to achieve immortality, by which is meant living as long as your particular body is capable of living — not becoming a god. According to Taoism, health and happiness also have a *way*, a Tao, that can be known. Study of this question by many people over thousands of years has revealed that the way to live healthier, happier, and longer, is to practice meditation and tai chi.

## 1.8
## What is the relationship between Taoism and tai chi?

Taoism is a scientific way of studying nature that tries to answer why things are the way they are. It tries to discover the principles of life. The *Tao Te Ching*, for example, explored the social and political interactions of humans. Tai chi does the same thing for fighting. Tai chi chuan is a system of fighting based on the Taoist inquiry into best fighting practices. The basic idea of tai chi is the principle of *yin* and *yang*, which is used as its symbol. The principle of *yin* and *yang* means that everything in the universe has its complement, its opposite; every action has its reaction. *Yang* means a strong force, hard. *Yin* represents a responding yielding force, soft. In the universe, the sun is *yang* and moon is *yin*; males are *yang* and females are *yin*. In any interaction you need two people, two objects, two forces. Tai chi is based on that realization and applying the principle of *yin* and *yang* in martial art. Accordingly, if someone attacks you with a *yang* force and you counter with a *yang* force, then the stronger will win — simple physics. You can rely on a *yang* force in all situations if you are the strongest person in the universe. In reality, there will always be someone stronger. However, to a *yang* attack you can always be *yin*. This is the idea of tai chi, to be *yin* to an attack. Thus, if you yield to an attack, meaning you bend to it and allow the attack to be exhausted, then you can counterattack just when your opponent is most exposed (and you won't need much strength to do so). Tai chi is the art of understanding the attack so as to respond, often by using the attack's power (see chapter 3 below).

## 1.9
## So, is tai chi standardized?

In the millennium since Chang San-feng, many variations and styles have developed naturally as the art was transmitted from teacher to student. It passed through many generations in the Chen village until members of the Yang family began to teach it publicly. Their style is called the Yang Style but there are also the Chen, Sun and Wu styles. Each styles is so named for the family who propagated that style. A style consists of the order of the movements that a particular master taught to his students, who in turn taught others. So maybe in the future there will be a 'Chu style'. In any event, each style is tai chi.

No matter the style, there are basic tai chi principles. These principles have been laid down by many old masters in the tai chi classics, which are included in *Tai Chi Chuan Principles & Practice* (*TCCP&P*). I also explain the principles and demonstrate the movements of the Yang style form on a DVD. By way of example, take Single Whip: if you change your height while doing the move (that is, the hips sink toward the ground or your head gets closer to the ceiling; that is, you move up or down), you are not doing tai chi. Correctly, you must stay at the same height; you must keep your pelvis tucked under. Generally, a common cause of incorrect tai chi is that they the body is too stiff or even rigid. Another major mistake concerns foot power: the heel must not move as you pivot. However, if you do tai chi incorrectly you will still improve your health. But it goes without saying: the more correctly you do tai chi, the more benefit you will get. It doesn't really matter which particular style you're doing — if you adhere to the basic principles, you are doing correct tai chi. So aspiring students should look for a teacher who follows the principles.

### 1.10
### Is Yang the most popular style because it is the easiest to learn?

First, no tai chi style is more difficult than any other, and it is never easy to attain high-level skills or mastery in any style. Yang style is popular because the Yang family was the first to teach tai chi to the public in Beijing. Furthermore, Yang Cheng-fu, the grandson of the founder of Yang style tai chi, traveled all over China, which also helped to popularize the style.

### 1.11
### Has tai chi been refined over the years?

Yes. To me, tai chi is like a rough gem. Throughout history, all the tai chi masters have polished the form, making the gem better and better. This is why I try to understand the old masters' teachings and piece them together. I also try to add my own insights into tai chi with my writing as well as my teaching. The reason is this: like the Taoists of old, I treat tai chi like a science and science always moves forward. It can always give us a better understanding. Science is the study of nature and tai chi is the study of the nature of the human body in terms of movement and self-defense.

### 1.12
### What are the tai chi classics?
### Is the *Tao Te Ching* a tai chi classic?

Luckily, many tai chi masters wrote down their insights. These writings gathered together are the canon of tai chi, simply referred to as the tai chi classics. Unfortunately, they do not give too many details about how to move the body but they give the principles to apply. They include "The Tai Chi Chuan Treatise," "The Song of the Thirteen Movements," and "Yang Cheng-fu's Ten Important Points." You can find my translations of the classics in Part Two of *Tai Chi Chuan Principles & Practice*. The *Tao Te Ching* is not a book on martial arts. As mentioned above, the *Tao Te Ching* is the quintessential statement of Taoist philosophy. It is the basis of the science of self-cultivation, health, and fighting technique known as tai chi. Reading the tai chi classics by themselves will not teach you how to do the form. You can only learn the form from a teacher. The classics will tell you how to move correctly as well as the theory of applying tai chi in combat. But again, a layman or tai chi novice cannot just pick up a classic and understand it on his or her own — you need a teacher. In the classics is the philosophy of fighting: how to overcome the opponent, and how to advance, retreat, and yield; as well as the principles of correct movement like the meaning of rooting, aligning the body, hard and soft, *yin* and *yang*. And the classics are based on Taoism and the *Tao Te Ching*.

### 1.13
### What is tai chi's place in the history of martial arts?

Tai Chi is, I believe, the highest evolution of martial arts because it does not emphasize force against force, but rather yielding and responding. In addition, tai chi movements actually heal the body. By way of contrast, the external martial arts make the body burn out because that training puts mileage on the body. As a healing exercise, tai chi often attracts practitioners who have long practiced external martial arts but, at some point, are unable to summon the energy for it. They are burned out and aged; tai chi is rejuvenating. Many who study external arts for a long time turn to tai chi to recover. Some of tai chi's most famous proponents and teachers came to tai chi for healing. I would also mention that the tai chi classics are often quoted but without attribution. Take Bruce Lee, perhaps the most famous martial artist in the world. His philosophy of fighting and movement has utilized the tai chi classics. So tai chi is not just the highest evolution of martial art but also a means of rejuvenating and improving martial arts in general.

### 1.14
### When did tai chi come to the United States? Who brought it?

I can't be certain about a first teacher of tai chi in the United States. But, to my knowledge, among the first to popularize tai chi in the United States was a woman named Sophia Delza (1903-1996). Prompted by a back injury that brought her professional dancing to an end, she studied tai chi with Ma Yueh-liang in Shanghai. Back in New York, she taught Wu style tai chi as movement and exercise, not a martial art. As a matter of fact, she even wrote to *T'ai Chi Magazine* saying she had never heard of tai chi as a self-defense practice and her teacher had never mentioned self-defense applications. She wrote a book, *T'ai Chi Ch'uan: Body And Mind In Harmony, An Ancient Way Of Exercise To Achieve Health And Tranquility* (1961). She also wrote magazine articles about tai chi and its health benefits. The person often credited as the first to popularize tai chi in the United States is Cheng Man-Ch'ing (1902-1975). A noted scholar, poet, and painter, he studied tai chi with Yang Cheng-fu. Interestingly, Man-Ch'ing contracted a lung disease and used tai chi to recover from it. Man-Ch'ing came to New York in 1964 and began teaching tai chi. Unfortunately, for the purposes of popularization and dissemination, since he didn't speak English he had to depend on interpreters to teach the art. As a result, he taught very few students directly and many of his principles were misinterpreted due, in part, to the language barrier. Man-Ch'ing's tai chi was very good but too many people claim to have been his students and few who make this claim really understand his teachings. Regardless, Robert Smith's book, *T'ai-chi: The "Supreme Ultimate" Exercise for Health, Sport, and Self-Defense* (1967), with Man-Ch'ing, made tai chi as well as Man-Ch'ing popular. Man-Ch'ing's "Yang-Style Tai Chi in 37 Postures" (commonly called the short form) is the first form students learn at my school. On the topic of early teachers of tai chi in this country, mention must be made of William C.C. Chen of Taiwan, who studied with Man-Ch'ing. Chen opened his own school here in New York early on (1965). He is one of the few people who teach tai chi fighting applications and his students win open tournaments.

## 1.15
### What does "lineage" mean in martial arts?

Until recently, martial arts were a necessary part of daily life for individual self-protection or for the protection of a whole village in times of societal unease. Obviously, those successful at defense had an edge in such times and did not want their techniques known. Skilled martial artists could attain fame and fortune, including recognition and even a professional position from the Emperor of China. Therefore, they closely guarded the knowledge of their skills and taught them only to family members or neighbors. Since only the members of a certain family knew a technique, it had to be learned from them. Over the last two centuries, as secret styles began to be taught to outsiders, the notion of lineage developed. Masters of a style would impart their secrets to a select few and designate them as heirs, masters of that style. Therefore, lineage is like a "family tree" of a particular style and to claim lineage is a teacher's way of claiming to be a member of a family's style, even if he or she is not genetically related to that family, and an authentic practitioner of that particular style. While not as transparent as a university system that awards degrees, lineage has been the way in which martial arts was handed down over time.

## 1.16
### What is your lineage?

Lineage is not as important as people make it out to be. I think the true practice of tai chi depends on a thorough understanding of the tai chi principles as well as a lot of practice. As an art and a science, you do not need to be bound by the expectations of a specific "family" and their idiosyncrasies. Making claims about lineage, boasting about ancestry, or showing-off certificates from famous masters, does not make you a good practitioner of tai chi, nor does it guarantee that you will be a good teacher. Even if you studied with Yang Cheng-fu himself, that does not mean you are as good as him. At the moment, there isn't a transparent, university-style system for certifying tai chi masters. My "lineage" is much like the 95% of tai chi practitioners around the world — Yang style. I learned tai chi from a student of Tung Ying-chieh (who was a student of Yang Cheng-fu) and I also learned from a Wu-style master (Wu style is an offshoot of the Yang style). Growing up in Hong Kong, I studied other martial arts styles as well. In this country, I learned Chen

Man-Ch'ing's 37-movement short form from William CC Chen. Mastering tai chi depends on self-cultivation over a long time and good teachers facilitate, this but they do not make it happen, no matter what their lineage.

While the history of tai chi is unclear (as noted above), it is certain that from the seventeenth century to the early nineteenth century, tai chi was a guarded secret of the Chen village. In the early nineteenth century, Yang Lu-shan (1799-1872) gained access to the village and learned tai chi. He is considered the father of the Yang style because he was the first to teach tai chi publicly. He was also known as Yang Wu Di, Invincible Yang, because he was never defeated in a fight (see *TCCP&P* pp. 4-5). His grandson, Yang Chang-fu (1883-1936), furthered this popularization of tai chi by traveling all over China with his students to demonstrate tai chi. He is the one who developed the tai chi form (called the long form) that nearly all people perform when they do tai chi today. In the mid-twentieth century, Chen Man-Ch'ing (1902-1975), student of Yang Chang-Fu, simplified the form into a 37-movement form. As I point out in my DVD, his form has 65 movements if each movement is counted. In my school, students learn the 65-movement short form before learning the long form. After the communist revolution in China, the government recognized the value of tai chi gathered tai chi masters from around China and asked them to devise a simplified form shorn of its martial application that people could do for health. They devised a 24-movement form that is done on both sides (for a total of 48 movements).

Recently, I saw footage of Tung Ying-chieh (1898-1961) posted online. Tung is reputed to be the best of Yang Cheng-fu's students and, therefore, seeing footage of Tung is the closest we can come to seeing tai chi as it was performed in the days of Cheng-fu. I was pleased to see that my study and practice of tai chi had made my form look like Tung's. In the footage, you can clearly see him exhibiting tai chi principles, like tucking in and leaning forward, that few tai chi practitioners understand today.

Tai chi should be done a certain way (with its fighting application in mind) because it works for fighting and for health. It works in terms of body alignment, power, and well-being. My approach is Taoist and true, I believe, to the spirit of Yang Lu-shan's efforts to teach tai chi to everyone. As in science, where the progress of one scientist depends on the past with Newton standing on the shoulders of Galileo, I stand on the shoulders of my teachers and the classics. I know there are a lot of rumors and misunderstandings about tai chi due in part to the mystique of lineages — with "my teacher did it this way" taking the place of comprehension. In what follows I will explain things as best I can and people can make their own judgment for this generation and many to come. In kung fu, everyone thinks their style is the best, tai chi is no exception to this. Everyone gets at least some things right but we should all be striving to do tai chi more correctly, and drop the bad habits, in order to get more benefit. Unfortunately, we don't have any photographs or videos of Lu-shan. We do have photographs of Cheng-fu and a couple films of Tung. More visual documentation of the old masters would be wonderful to have, for it would clear up many questions. Still, we can use a Taoist, scientific approach, in our tai chi practice and do the best we can, leaving out the personal politics. Meaning, we train according to the tai chi principles and the science of correct body alignment. Hopefully, my book will help toward that end.

### 1.17
### How does a Taoist school differ from a karate school?

Tai Chi Chuan comes from Taoism and success in tai chi depends upon a Taoist approach. The Taoist approach to life is relaxed: a person should do what he or she does and derive enjoyment from that. If life is not enjoyable, something is wrong somewhere. Obviously, the Taoist approach is different from the hard style systems. Many hard style systems are militaristic with a master as a sergeant and students as soldiers. If the student fails to execute a move correctly, he or she may be punished in some way. But tai chi doesn't work that way. It is like singing: you cannot force someone to sing if he doesn't want to sing; further, you can't force someone to sing a happy song if he is not happy. Likewise, a person can't be forced to do tai chi. To do good tai chi, you must be very relaxed and so the atmosphere of my school is very relaxed. There is no bullying but rather a spirit of cooperation in which students help each other improve themselves. Here, the students are all brothers and sisters, which is a Taoist idea. For that reason, there is no hierarchy or any kind of belt and rank system at CK Chu Tai Chi. Students come here to help each other cultivate themselves mentally and physically. Moreover, instruction in my school is one-to-one because each person needs to learn tai chi at his or her own pace. Here our goal is not to please the drill sergeant but to help people discover their true selves through realization of true alignment and yielding.

CK Chu Tai Chi does offer a certification program for those students who need or who desire additional structure to guide their study of tai chi. In the old days, students would live with a master for 20 years or more as part of his family before leaving and taking on his or her own students. Such arrangements are not very practical in today's world, and yet the system of belts, as in karate, creates hierarchy. That is contrary to Taoist ideals. This program is intended to provide an incentive for students to reach higher levels in their practice. The program is modeled on the university system and awards credit hours to those enrolled in the program. As part of the curriculum, students also meet with me one-on-one. The series of four certificates recognize a student's personal evolution toward a goal of better practice over several years.

### 1.18
### What is the correct curriculum of tai chi chuan?

Tai Chi Chuan is a fighting art and requires a healthy body and sound mind. A proper curriculum includes four disciplines, which serve as pillars to the house of study that is practicing tai chi. The student should work on these disciplines every day: the tai chi form, *chi kung*, *nei kung*, and meditation. On top of these pillars comes advanced training in the art of tai chi: push-hands, fighting applications, and weapons training. For example, at CK Chu Tai Chi, there are continual and ongoing classes in tai chi, *Eternal Spring*, *Nei Kung*, Push-Hands, Fighting, and Meditation. Periodically, classes in weapons and Taoist philosophy are also given.

Depending on student interest, CK Chu Tai Chi also trains fighters for tournaments. Over the years, my school has trained many champions of open full-contact tournaments. Their training begins with the four pillars. Most students are not interested in fighting competitively but they are interested in healing. They study the same basic curriculum to achieve better health. Tai chi training meets the needs of all ages and health needs.

# II. TAI CHI & HEALTH

## 2.1
## What is the definition of health in your view?

Being healthy not only means the absence of sickness: it also means developing the ability to use our unique bodies and minds to their fullest potential. Tai chi makes the body strong, integrated and coordinated, so that it can move gracefully, quickly and powerfully. Tai chi also promotes the development of a healthy mind, which allows us to see into the essence of life, and to think critically, imaginatively, and creatively.

Health of body and health of mind are inseparable. Healthy people are full of positive energy and confidence. Their body's senses are keener. They feel strong and ready to take on any activity they choose — be it running, jumping, or catching a ball. Age doesn't slow them down. Healthy people embody eternal youthfulness, even in old age; and, just like young children, healthy people feel that everything is well and there is nothing to worry about.

With a healthy body and mind, goals can be seen clearly and attained easily. Then, people are able to make the correct decisions for their personal paths and their achievement of happiness. An unhealthy body limits the potential for happiness by imposing constant limitations, placing a person at the mercy of ill health. An unhealthy mind cannot think clearly, and may make incorrect decisions that can ultimately cause harm.

## 2.2
## How can tai chi help me achieve good health?

Every day, it seems, there is a new report confirming the health benefits of tai chi whether for arthritis, stress, fibromyalgia, or other problems. Today's science is verifying that the Taoist practice of tai chi is a way of health. Practicing tai chi strengthens the entire body from the bones to the muscles and from the cell to the organs because it improves your body's alignment, flexibility, coordination, and functioning. In turn, this improves blood and lymph circulation while it massages the organs and bodily systems. With an improved posture and a healthier internal arrangement of your components, a regenerative and replenishing flow of *chi*, your vital energy or "life force," will flow through you. Tai chi heals and charges the body up, making us feel good afterwards — not drained.

Through exercises that align the body, tai chi practitioners gain more balance and coordination they use in their daily lives. Also, tai chi emphasizes the improvement of tendons and bones over muscles so the body becomes more dense and stronger as a whole unit. Breathing is a central concern in tai chi. By consciously improving breathing capacity through exercise the tai chi way, practitioners begin to breathe deeply all the time — not just during the form. This deep breathing helps tai chi practitioners be their levelheaded best in their daily lives.

Finally, tai chi also builds mind-body connection, something calisthenics and sports training do not do. By fostering of relaxation, tai chi improves mental health so that you can be more yourself. In addition, by training to integrate the mind and body, the mind stops wasting *chi* on worry or negative thinking so that *chi* can be used for healing past emotional trauma, physical injury, or for other positive things. Tai chi (this includes *chi kung, nei kung*, the tai chi form, push-hands, and *san shou* or fighting) exercises the whole body as one piece so that you can be the best 'You' — the best mentally, physically, and emotionally. Tai chi, then, is a true maintenance system for the whole body.

## 2.3
## Why should I do tai chi instead of some other "maintenance" program?

In strictly mechanical terms, the major goal of tai chi is the development of correct alignment, posture and balance. When the body's joints are properly aligned, and when muscles and tendons are properly conditioned to maintain good posture, the organs and tissues of the body are naturally supplied with a healthy amount of blood and *chi*. Imagine, for a moment, a garden hose snaking through the garden without kinks in it — water flows smoothly and quietly within. Now put a loose kink in the hose, what happens to the water? Even a loose kink will slow the water and cause it to make an angry noise inside the hose. Tighten the kink it harder and what happens? The flow of water can be stopped altogether by a tight kink. Good alignment, like a garden hose without kinks, allows a greater and more stable flow of blood and *chi* through the body. But wear and tear, daily stress, injury, and misalignment are all kinks in your *chi* irrigation system. How will you fix this?

When people think of "getting in shape," they usually have the image of the body-builder with bulging muscles in mind or they have been convinced that good health means a specific type of "cardio" workout, like "jazzercise". If a person joins a gym, you can play around doing sports, like tennis or basketball, or indeed do aerobics. Those are good exercises for meeting people, hanging out with friends, and blowing off steam. If a person is more serious-minded and consults a trainer at a club, the typical exercise program he or she will get will be concerned with building up muscles in isolation from the body for aesthetic purposes and perhaps have a "cardio" goal of running a certain number of laps and so fort. This type of fitness training is better than nothing and some of it can be complementary to tai chi, but it is very superficial. For example, going to the gym might make you breathe harder for a short period of time, but once you are done, you resume your shallow breathing. What then have you gained?

Tai chi is a scientific approach to improving the body's health so that when you are old, you are not infirm. Two key differences come to mind when thinking about going to the gym vs. doing tai chi: development of the mind and development of the breath. In the gym or while doing sports-based exercise, the mind is stressed by having to win all the time, rather than connect with the body. In tai chi, practitioners learn how to give the mind a break and thereby free up the energy the mind uses for healing purposes (see 7.16). Furthermore, tai chi teaches you how to "put the mind inside the body," meaning, to erase the separation of mind-body so that you can be one whole entity, one whole 'You.' Tai chi does this because it does not contain the stress of goal-oriented sports or fitness programs. Because tai chi emphasizes the integration of the entire body (with mind) within a single unit, it is more effective than working on an individual muscle for fostering overall health. For example, when catching a ball the "tai chi way", the entire body moves like a coordinated, well-oiled machine, without putting excess strain on any particular body part. The goal of tai chi is proper body alignment so that those kinks will be removed and the *chi* will flow. Crucial to this process is the development of proper breathing.

When working out at the gym, breathing is a necessity, of course, but never a focus. Rather, you breathe at the gym while doing activities and your breathing merely lifts and expands the rib cage to give the lungs room to expand upward. While this increases the amount of oxygen entering the body and carbon dioxide leaving, it does little else. Moreover, the benefits to the lungs occurring during exercise do not carryover into the rest of life, and after jogging or aerobics class people return to their shallow breathing habits. In tai chi, breathing comes from the diaphragm. Such breathing maximizes gas exchange by allowing the lungs to expand downward, which in turn massages the digestive organs in the abdomen. The digestive organs, in turn, work better. Through tai chi training, diaphragm breathing becomes second nature and the body begins to breathe this way all the time, making a person who trains this way more relaxed and more efficient in their activities.

## 2.4
## What is *chi*?

In my opinion, *chi* is part of the electromagnetic wave spectrum. This spectrum includes all the possible waves that can exist from the very long radio wave to the very tiny gamma ray. Visible light is a tiny portion of this spectrum. This tiny portion of visible light is from red to violet. Human eyes cannot see wavelengths that are longer or shorter than that range, like infrared (longer) or ultraviolet (shorter) respectively. But some insects can see ultraviolet waves, and scientists have developed instruments to see infrared light, as in night vision goggles. I point this out to show that something that seems invisible to the naked eye is visible to other organisms or to humans only with the aid of special devices.

Our body wave or *chi* is slightly above infrared, just below the radar (or micro) wave. As you know, a microwave oven produces microwaves inside a chamber in which you put your food. This food heats up because the microwaves excite the water molecules in the food. Like microwaves, *chi* excites the body's molecules and creates heat. So, the wavelength of *chi* must be close to the microwave range, perhaps from a fraction of a millimeter to a millimeter long.

### 2.5
### Can the amount of *chi* be measured?

Yes, it could be, but no instrument currently exists that is capable of such a measurement. Such a device would be a cross between a brain wave detector and a heat detector. When practicing *nei kung* or meditation, a person notices heat traveling through the body. Such occurrences could be measured and compared with the body's *chi* state before and after practice. It would be a good idea for the scientific community to invent a *chi*-measuring instrument. I'm surprised such an instrument does not exist yet. After all, we can measure a brain wave and that is the same kind of thing.

### 2.6
### Could you elaborate on the role of *chi* in the body —
### the way it works, how it becomes obstructed,
### and how tai chi improves *chi* in the body?

*Chi*, in short, is the 'life force.' Everyone has *chi* in every part of the body — if you didn't, you would not be alive. Everyday use of the body wears it down, like putting miles on a car, weakening the amount of *chi* in the body and obstructing *chi* flow. Without maintenance, those miles will add up to fatigue, illness, or disease. In order to maintain the body and mitigate the impact of all those miles, *chi* needs to circulate to replenish and regenerate the whole body system. When the *chi* is strong, the body is strong and every part of the body functions properly. If *chi* is weak, problems will accrue; for example, weak *chi* in the heart leads to heart problems in time; *chi* not going to the kidney will lead to kidney problems in time. If *chi* remains weak, the body cannot regenerate, ward off disease, or function properly, so it will wear down, or age, faster. Tai chi increases the amount of *chi* available to the body and by improving the body's alignment improves the circulation of the increased *chi* to all the parts of the body so that the whole body can regenerate and replenish. The better the alignment and the better the circulation of *chi*, the more *chi* there will be — this will improve the alignment and the circulation of *chi* and so on.

For example, over my years of teaching, quite a few students have come to my school, seeking relief from 'headaches' and migraines. A headache, in my experience, results from the blockage of *chi*. Many students have gained relief from doing one or two classes of *Eternal Spring* because *chi kung* improves the circulation of *chi*; it works out the kinks in the hose that caused the pain of the headache (see also 2.19).

### 2.7
### What is alignment and why is it so important?

Whether sitting, that is static, or moving around, that is dynamic, gravity pulls on the body causing stress. Poor posture causes stress to the body, and if not corrected will cause pain. Good posture is only possible if the skeleton is lined up correctly: this is alignment. The circulation of *chi* improves, as discussed in the previous question, with improved alignment.

People spend a lot of time in static positions. They sit for a long time on sofas or easy chairs. Sitting there, the body has to support itself while gravity continues to pull on it. Say you are sitting on a sofa, your head lolling back, and your back apparently resting on the cushions. Well, certain parts of the body have to hold you in that lazy pose and those parts are being stressed. This stress over a long period of time (a few hours a day, everyday, every year . . . ) will cause problems because the parts of the body supporting the lazy pose are not getting sufficient *chi*. Why? They were not made to support your body in such a position. The outcome is blocked *chi* flow, and people feel this as pain — perhaps immediately upon getting up, or, much later when you happen to bend over, long after getting up. Or take reading: in this static activity, the head leans and drops down causing stress to your shoulders; neck pain will develop in due course. The sources of pain are numerous and include those resulting from computer work, carrying bags always on one side, standing while on the subways holding the rail, etc. But they can be as simple as being tall inside architecture designed for shorter heights, requiring you to constantly stoop. Stooping, as in reading, will lead to tightness and pain in the neck and shoulder area.

For the body to move correctly, the frame (the skeleton, tendons, and muscles) must be balanced so that the stress of movement falls on the appropriate part of the body. *Chi kung* and *nei kung* train the muscles and tendons to align your frame properly and keep it in a proper alignment. These exercise regimens give you a foundation for proper execution of the tai chi form. Moreover, tai chi is like moving *chi kung* and *nei kung*. Doing the form, in other words, also improves your alignment. For example, a common problem people have is tight hips, which causes the knees to cave in (bend towards each other) when they are bent. The result is disrupted *chi* flow because the body is misaligned and off balance. People can be born with alignment problems, or acquire them through injury or bad habits, such as always carrying a bag on one side. Whatever the source of the problem, tai chi training is a process of bringing the body into alignment so that your *chi* will circulate better and you will be a healthier, happier person. That is why alignment is important.

## 2.8
## Is tai chi good for people with back and knee problems?

Yes. Before elaborating, it is important to note a few things. Earlier, it was mentioned that the body is put out of alignment by daily activities. While it is true that sedentary habits put the body out of alignment, and it goes without saying that sports injuries or ankle sprains do too, the body may have started life out of alignment. People can be born with imperfect alignment — toes that go too far out or too far in, knees that buckle in, flat feet, and a whole host of other congenital imperfections. In some ways, the body is what the body is, but it can also be made into the best body. Indeed, it surprises many people that the famous Bruce Lee was a very weak child. He remained weak until he decided to make himself as fit as possible. This involved diet, exercise, and mental development. Imperfections from birth can be corrected, weaknesses strengthened, alignment improved. If these imperfections and misalignments are ignored, and, for example, you walk on a poorly aligned leg, then your posture will worsen and your health will decline.

How is this done? Consider the body as a building. Buildings need to have a solid foundation or they will lean. In 2008, I visited the famous Leaning Tower of Pisa where, purportedly, groundbreaking experiments in physics were performed long ago. Now, engineers struggle just to hold the building up. The building does not sit on solid ground and even during construction it listed, so the builder actually tried to hide the list by curving the structure. This worked for a time, and it made it seem as though the leaning wasn't so bad. But gravity has had a few hundred years to pull on a misaligned, improperly maintained, and poorly located building. The result is that without sophisticated propping mechanisms, the tower will fall. The pyramids in Egypt, on the other hand, are among the world's oldest structures and because they are aligned well, they will never tip over. They are built with, shall we say, a tai chi stance: a firm, wide base narrowing to a tip. Likewise, tai chi aims to rebuild the body from the root up.

The knees and the back are very important and the use of them for the duration of life is very desirable, so it is important to do exercises that keep them healthy. People are born with a crooked spine and with all the sitting people do, gravity pulls on the back in the wrong way, causing pain. The spine is supposed to be able to twist — if you do not twist and loosen the spine, you will get arthritis and backaches. Another problem with the back comes from lifting objects that are too heavy, or lifting incorrectly. Often, you see people wearing thick leather belts. They do that for the same reason engineers have propped up the tower in Pisa — so they can still do the job even though their body can't. Tai chi repairs the back because it places the body in correct alignment. This means the spine is suspended from the top of the head like a string of loose beads that are free to twist and turn. The twisting and turning in tai chi strengthens the spine and the muscles and tendons holding the spine in place. This type of correct alignment and correct movement will stimulate the blood and *chi* circulation and heal the back. Align the body correctly, treat the body properly (for example, don't lift a piano if you are not Superman), and lift with the whole body — from the feet, with the legs. A healthy body does not need an artificial support such as the weightlifter's belt.

In general, your back and knees should be coordinated during most of the body's movements. For example, when your knees bend, your lower back should not be arched (for a diagram of proper alignment, see *The Book of Nei Kung,* p. 23). The knees should move in a linear motion. Like your finger, your knees should not be twisted. It's the back and knee linking together that gives you balance and rootedness in tai chi. Lack of this coordination can cause back pain.

In all tai chi movements, the whole body should move as one unit. A particularly important movement found in *Eternal Spring, nei kung,* and the tai chi form, is the Horse Stance. This exercise fixes the back, improves the coordination between the knee and the back, and circulates the *chi,* among many other benefits. The key is to do the exercise correctly, toes slightly pointed in, knees out, back round. But follow the tai chi principles, and all of tai chi improves the back and knee. For example, in Heel Kick, the hands, chest, back, and leg are coordinated and moving as one unit with rootedness and striking power. Do it correctly and do it on a regular basis, and you will be healthier.

## 2.9
## What is the importance of flexibility and coordination to health?

As a person ages, the body gets tighter and stiffer. Like a rubber band, if you don't use it, it dries out, becomes brittle, and breaks. But if you use it as intended and don't over-stretch it, the rubber band will stay rubbery and elastic. You have to work your body to keep it rubbery. If you don't, your body will become increasingly stiff and the tendons will tighten. Stiffness in the body, particularly in the joints, results from those parts of the body not getting enough *chi.* Now you risk injury at any time — step wrong on the stairs and break your ankle. Tai chi pulls the skeleton, tendons, and muscles into the right places to keep the body elastic. It works the joints (neck, back, knees, wrist, etc.) keeping them lubricated and mobile so they can withstand certain pressures. Someone who does tai chi can trip or step wrong but their ankle will just bounce back, just like a little child's ankle — maybe stinging a little. It won't shatter as would an ankle with osteoporosis. It is the difference between the young sapling bending in the wind and the old tree snapping apart. By doing tai chi, the joints receive plenty of *chi,* which keeps the body flexible.

Organisms operate as whole bodies: the whale or the cat do not function as just minds or just bodies, nor do they function just as a tail and a head. Like them, humans must function as a whole body. This involves coordination between the mind and the body as well as coordination between the various systems of the body. In modern society, too often the parts are dealt with separately and emotional problems are never connected to bodily ailments. But the body, the person as a whole, must be healthy as a whole, and that is the aim of tai chi. When catching a ball, playing soccer, juggling, any kind of fighting, or just getting through the day, you need to coordinate your whole body to interact with objects and other people. The body and mind must be coordinated. Tai chi, as a fighting art, studies coordination for martial purposes but this same study can improve your coordination in any aspect of life. Some people shy away from the martial aspects of tai chi, but it is a martial art. All animals defend themselves; to be fully human — to be able to use your body and mind in coordination — you should know how to fight. Alignment and flexibility are at their maximum in a properly coordinated and executed strike: knowing how to do this is the only way to get the full benefit from the tai chi form, since each movement is a fighting move.

### 2.10
### What effect does tai chi, *chi kung*, and *nei kung*, have on the body?

It is not how much you eat but how much you assimilate that matters. We know the body takes energy from the food we eat, but it needs to transform that food into *chi*, an energy the body can utilize. The body then needs to distribute the *chi* efficiently throughout the system so that it can stay healthy or heal itself. *Chi* is distributed throughout the body through meridians, the body's irrigation system. Without proper conversion and distribution, food, water, and air can do little for our bodies. What's more, if the meridians are obstructed in any way, the *chi* will not flow.

Tai chi, *chi kung*, and *nei kung* support the process of transformation and distribution. Exercising the body according to these regimens creates and maintains proper alignment of the bones, muscles, and tendons. While doing the exercises, one can actually feel a realignment taking place, especially in the areas of old injuries. Improving alignment allows the meridians to move *chi*. When energy is transformed well and is circulated in the form of *chi*, it heals the internal organs and systems, including the kidneys and the heart. Correct body alignment is an absolute necessity if the meridians are to be open and free flowing.

Local pain in the body indicates injury or blockage to a specific area of the meridian system and is thus a call for attention. A migraine, for instance, occurs because there is a blockage. Doing tai chi and *nei kung* can eliminate it. By the way, excessive worrying will short-circuit the *chi*. It is like crossing positive and negative electrical terminals. By worrying, one wastes the *chi*.

### 2.12
### What is the problem with sports-based exercise?

There is nothing wrong with it at all. If you just want to move around, sweat, listen to tunes, and you enjoy the exercise, then go for it. After all, socializing and having fun is good for health — so is bowling with friends and playing volleyball. But those exercises are not designed to improve your alignment or maintain your body's functions.

## 2.13
## How does running compare with tai chi?

Running is an exercise with only one dimension. It is good cardiovascular exercise and better than doing nothing, but running is not a whole body health system. Running as an exercise is the performance of repetitive motion. Many people overdo running and get hurt because they continue the repetition over too long a time on a body with alignment problems and end up causing strain to the body. A little bit of running is good for the body and you should get out and 'stretch your legs.' However, excessive running taxes the body. It puts stress on the knees, hipbones and joints. It ages the body faster, making it stiff. In my opinion, running has many limitations. Running is like putting miles on a car without proper maintenance and care. That car will age fast and quickly stop working.

## 2.14
## What about weightlifting?

The same is true of weightlifting as of running. It has only one dimension — it just builds strength in specific areas. It does not build the body as a whole. Rather, certain movements are done with weight to work, and thus build, certain muscles. Real health and power come from moving the body as one piece — like an animal. That is, using muscle groups with other muscle groups and those muscles together with the skeleton, lungs, mind, etc. — the whole body as one unit. In my opinion, Mr. Universe-type weightlifting makes the body muscle-bound and less flexible. Such people have difficulty unbending their arms all the way for example. If you build up muscles to lift 400 lbs in one direction, that same built-up muscle will hinder other muscles from working. So, just because a weightlifter can pick up a heavy object doesn't mean he can deliver a solid punch. In the sports world, bodies are developed to suit the specific requirements of the activity. Weightlifters bulk up but you won't find a bulky swimmer or a bulky basketball player. Both of the latter are sleek and trim because they have to move their whole body. Look at Michael Phelps — 14 Olympic gold medals so far. He doesn't look the least bit muscle-bound but he is very strong.

Of course, a little weightlifting can be useful if you are weak, but be sure to use free weights and not machines. Machines just provide linear motion. You want the whole body to be involved during any exercise. You also want to include the mind. Both running and weightlifting exclude the mind. In both sports, you can escape the stress of the everyday. You have a bad day and go for an eight-mile run or go to the gym, crank up the tunes, and lift. Both give you benefit because you need to be able to take a break from life's stresses. But in both, you are divorcing the mind from the body — using the muscle memory of the repetitive motion to let the mind go off and daydream or zone out. This is not as beneficial as tai chi's integration of mind and body to improve and heal the whole. Also, the other exercises just discussed do not increase your *chi* nor will they teach you self-defense.

## 2.15
### Besides using light weights, what are some exercises other than tai chi for strengthening the body?

Tai chi is the best exercise for strengthening the body, but some people may wish to do other exercises in conjunction with tai chi. In that case, traditional exercises like push-ups, sit-ups, chin-ups, swimming, mountain climbing, hiking, jumping rope, and jogging are highly recommended. They are all good exercise. Other activities are also good, like skateboarding, ice-skating, skiing, basketball, etc. but they are all limited. They are only bad if you overdo it or if you body is not up to doing it at all. But I do not recommend bodybuilding per se, because that just works on individual muscles and does not work on the body as a whole. Also, a lot of people get hurt doing it: for example, they try to lift too much or get carried away, take steroids, and ruin their kidneys. Anyway, these other exercises should only serve as a hobby, not a complete health regimen.

In general, people should do an exercise program of *chi kung*, tai chi form (slow and then fast), push-hands, fighting, weapons and sparring. I also recommend *nei kung*, meditation, iron palm training and body toughening and conditioning. This is a more complete exercise system than just push-ups or sit-ups and much more beneficial for your body.

## 2.16
### Does Yoga deliver benefits similar to tai chi?

There is nothing wrong with doing yoga or most other kinds of exercise. Today we are too sedentary, so if people increase their activity doing any exercise, that is a good thing. If everyone did tai chi too, that would be even better. Now, yoga is not a whole body health system either. It does not give you self-defense or whole body movement. It may help you to improve your alignment through increasing your flexibility. This alone makes it a good exercise for many people because they are inflexible and need stretching. But if you rely exclusively on yoga, then in time you may be able to twist the body into a pretzel shape but you will lose your elasticity — your bounce — as a result. For example, in my early years of teaching tai chi, I had a student who was in decent shape but he had a problem with tai chi. He just couldn't do the movements, couldn't hold the postures. Then, one day, he showed me his yoga exercise and how he could twist. Ah ha, I saw his body was overstretched and could not bounce back. He had lost his elasticity. So, yoga can be a phase of your health regimen, as can running and weightlifting. But don't overdo those exercises and practice tai chi as well.

Another problem with yoga is that it doesn't give you more *chi*. Doing yoga opens the body and this makes the *chi* flow a little better if you do it correctly. However, many people doing yoga just stretch the body one part at a time and sometimes people overdo the stretch on one part. This can cause misalignment and loss of elasticity in that one part of the body. Tai chi integrates the body into one solid, lively piece, so the whole body is alive. It is not linear, working just one muscle in one direction, nor does it try to stretch and twist one way and one way only. Finally, there is the matter of efficiency — spend a little time on tai chi, get a lot of benefit but spend a little time on yoga, get very little benefit. People tell me all the time that after just one class of *Eternal Spring* they feel energized — like a car after a tune up. But go to one yoga class and for the time spent on it, the body is not much different. Also, a lot of people injure themselves at their first or second yoga class because they are overzealous or the instruction is poor. They wind up hurt, and being hurt is not an improvement.

As you can see, tai chi is different in many ways. It works on the whole body and is about mind-body coordination. Tai chi works on the healing energy — the *chi*. By increasing *chi* and improving circulation, tai chi works on the internal organs, the breathing apparatus, and the energy of the whole body down to the cellular level. Its movements move the whole body as a system. It does not just exercise one muscle at a time. After practicing for a long time, tai chi can be used for self-defense and its philosophy of yielding — "use four ounces of power to deflect the force of a thousand pounds" — can serve you in everyday life. It is preventive health care that slows down the aging process. To me, there is no comparison to other exercise programs.

### 2.17
### Is it true that tai chi slows the aging process?

Definitely. Tai chi slows the aging process by making the body healthy and strong. The healthy body coincides with a positive mental outlook — life is enjoyable. A person with a healthy body and mind has an easier time making appropriate decisions while not having to struggle and fight to achieve goals.

Our main goal isn't to slow the aging process, but it is a bonus that results from our practice. Tai chi opens windows for your mental and physical health. Taoists call this ideal, this state of having the wisdom of age and the body of youth, "eternal spring."

### 2.18
### What are your views about consumption of supplements, medicine, and stimulants (especially alcohol or other chemicals, either prescribed or not)?

There is so much information out there about medicines, supplements and other substances that one can easily be confused and misled. Most of it has no solid scientific foundation. We are pretty much in a trial-and-error stage of the game. Many supplements on the market are modern-day snake oil created using pseudo-science.

I believe some of the information is legitimate and helpful, but the majority of it is just commercial advertisement. The manufacturers hire writers to promote their products in magazines and on TV, saying that doctors recommend them. Their messages can be quite misleading. This puts us, the consumers, in danger. We must protect ourselves from being harmed by things that are supposed to help us. We must educate ourselves, and learn to distinguish what is good from what is not.

As for myself, after looking into all arguments, I have come to believe that B vitamins, Vitamin C, and Vitamin E are good for me. I do not take any other supplement because I have not decided whether they are good or safe to take. They may have side effects. The body may not be able to absorb the nutrients. The company may not be reliable in delivering the promised quality. Why would I want to subject myself to something that might have negative effects?

Almost every packaged food item in American supermarkets carries a label that indicates the ingredients and the nutrition. The information is made available; yet, ours is one of the unhealthiest countries in the world. Americans tend to look for easy ways out of health problems. They take a pill for this, a pill for that. For me, it is more effective and enjoyable to do some tai chi, *chi kung*, *nei kung* and meditation. I always look forward to practicing and wish I had more time to do them all. I say, let us beat inertia and do something to strengthen our bodies. There are no quick fixes.

Now, a small amount of alcohol occasionally will not hurt us. However, one glass of wine per week is already too much because it takes a long time for the body to get it out of the system. One needs to do a lot of exercise to sweat it out.

To sustain health, it is best to stay away from chemicals and substances as much as possible. Obtain necessary nutrients from good, fresh food. A diet of vegetables, seafood and a small amount of meat will be good for us. Avoid canned food; processed vegetables have lost most of their nutrients. It is far better to get something fresh from the market and spend a few minutes cooking it.

My suggested formula for health is: eat fresh, quality food in a small amounts; do tai chi, *nei kung*, *chi kung*, and meditate daily. Finally, take B vitamins, C and E obtained from a reputable manufacturer.

### 2.19
### On page 84 of *Tai Chi Chuan Principles & Practice* you discuss postnatal and prenatal breathing. What is the difference between the two?

The postnatal breath is the normal breathing of air. The prenatal breath is the *chi*, the invisible life force that is inside the body and is the basis of acupuncture. In fact, ancient Chinese doctors mapped out the paths of the *chi* inside the body; these paths are called meridians. The gate to adjusting and controlling the *chi* is called the meridian point (also known as the acupuncture point).

The prenatal breath is associated more with the electromagnetic wave of *chi* than with the normal breathing air of ionized oxygen. I discuss *chi* in detail in an article titled "Invisible Light," published in *Qi Magazine* (volume 7, number 2, summer 1997), available free on my website (www.chutaichi.com) (see also *TCCP&P*, p. 139).

## 2.20
### What is the *tan tien* and what role, if any, does it have in tai chi?

According to the meridian theory of Traditional Chinese Medicine, there are three *tan tiens*: lower, middle, and upper. The lower *tan tien* (or "region of vital heat," often called the "reservoir of *chi*") is located a couple of inches below the navel and towards the spine (it is inside the body, not at the level of the skin). This area is your energy center, your *chi* reservoir, and the center of gravity of the body. The middle *tan tien* (or "crimson palace") is located below the heart; the upper *tan tien* ("third eye") is between and behind the eyebrows. Training *chi*, whether for *chi kung*, meditation, or martial arts, begins with the development of the lower *tan tien*. In fact, it is so fundamental that mention of *tan tien* in the martial arts refers to the lower *tan tien* (as is the case in this text).

There are two important points to the development of *chi* and the *tan tien*: breathing and moving from the *tan tien*. By breathing to the diaphragm (to the *tan tien*), you will fill the *chi* reservoir. Whenever you do a lot of *chi kung* and tai chi, this area is charged up, like a battery, and will feel warm to the touch. This heat signifies the generation of the macroscopic orbit (the term for the circulation of *chi* through a meridian leading out of the *tan tien* downwards and continuing around the body and up the back, over the head, and down the front of the body). To reach a higher level of tai chi, do all the movements from the *tan tien* to improve your *chi* flow. Moving from the *tan tien* means the hand's or foot's movement is not separate from the waist. It is just like jumping. When you jump you jump from the *tan tien*. Hold your fingers there and jump; you will feel the *tan tien* firms up first. In tai chi fighting positions, the same thing happens. The *tan tien* firms up by pushing against the floor through the body and back out and this force rebounds to be expressed through the hands. The power doesn't start form the ground but from the *tan tien*. I often use the analogy of the whip: the *tan tien* is the handle or your movement and when you flick that handle, the movement will be expressed in your extremities. Your hand, in other words, is the end of the whip that is flicked from the *tan tien*. A person in good health will feel lots of heat in the *lower tan tien* while practicing tai chi. To develop good health, learn to pay attention to this spot and learn to move from the *tan tien* (see questions 5.15, 6.5).

## 2.21
### Do we get a good cardiovascular workout from tai chi?

Yes. Doing tai chi slowly has cardiovascular benefits. As a matter of fact, the whole body — especially the lungs, the heart and the related body breathing system — is being worked when you do tai chi slowly. Slow tai chi warms up the body and expands and contracts the muscles so that you can tai chi faster later on without shock and wear-and-tear to the system.

It is a common misconception to think tai chi is only done slowly just because you see people practicing tai chi slowly in the park. This is only one phase of training.

As a matter of fact, doing tai chi slowly and with correct breathing is very difficult but very beneficial. The slower you do it the better. Later on, our goal is also to do tai chi as fast as possible. The faster we do the form, the greater the cardiovascular benefits there will be for the body. In fact, 30 minutes of fast form is more beneficial than 30 minutes of running. Running is only a one-dimensional exercise, whereas tai chi is an integrated, full body workout.

### 2.22
### Can you elaborate on how slow and fast tai chi affect bodily systems?

Doing the tai chi form slowly strengthens the muscles, tendons and breathing system and prepares you to do tai chi faster later on. If you do it fast right away, your breathing may not be smooth enough and you may injure yourself without knowing it. Your lungs are like balloons. If you blow up a balloon too fast, you may burst it. On the other hand, if you stretch the balloon before you blow it up, you will inflate the balloon more evenly. The same is true of the lungs. Doing the form slowly prepares your lungs for doing the fast form.

The benefits of slow and fast tai chi are, in a sense, unlimited. For example, when you do tai chi slowly, the *chi* will sink into the bones, work on the cellular level and increase bone density. Also, doing tai chi slowly trains your mind to adopt a meditative mindset.

When you do tai chi fast the mind is more alert, more attentive and more responsive. You are ready for anything. When tai chi is done fast, it works on the intrinsic animal instinct and fast reaction. In fact, most people ignore their animal characteristics. They think people are just intellectual and that "man is mind." Tai chi unifies the mind and the body.

Slow and fast tai chi develop a great sensitivity — the sixth sense, you could call it. This is one of the many benefits of tai chi but it's hard to explain to people.

### 2.23
### Can you elaborate on the benefits of doing the tai chi form slowly?

Through slow, deliberate movement, relaxation can be learned, and with relaxation comes healing of the body and mind. The more relaxed you are, the slower you can go and the more relaxed you become and the more healing occurs. So practicing the form slowly is a long term project with increasing benefits. Relaxation and speed are related. Ultimately, from this slowness will come speed. A person who is tense rushes through the form, whereas the more relaxed a person is, the slower he or she can go. So by seeming to do nothing, you achieve everything — this paradox is a basic principle of Taoism, the source of tai chi.

A central concept in the *Tao Te Ching* is *wu wei* as in the expression *"wu wei wu yao but wei,"* which means, "do nothing, yet nothing left undone" (*Chu Meditation,*

p. 70). As developed throughout the *Tao Te Ching*, the idea of *wu wei* is the contradiction that doing something apparently not useful or promoting anything (like yourself or your career) actually does something. Taoist meditation, for example, is the practice of doing nothing — just sitting still without moving and without thinking (see chapter 7). The result is a healthier body and brain. Besides charging your body up, your brain gets a rest from its ceaseless working so it too is recharged.

Ideally, the tai chi form should be done in a *wu wei* way; completely relaxed and without effort — no extra flourishes to the hands or any unnecessary movement of the shoulders. Tai chi movements are done correctly when the body's dynamic is without tension or force, as if doing nothing. Of course, doing the form without effort is very difficult and can only be done after a lot of practice, instruction, and correction. That too is *wu wei*: what looks effortless results from a lot of effort.

### 2.24
### So, does *wu wei* mean I can do the form however I want?

No, that is not the meaning of *wu wei*. The appearance of seeming to make no effort is actually the result of a great deal of effort. It is similar to the *yin-yang* principle — effort and effortlessness go together. In other words, as mentioned throughout this text, you must follow the tai chi principles to achieve the benefits of tai chi.

At first, to learn tai chi the body must be ordered to do certain things — the complete opposite of the ideal just described. Tai chi is a science that, if followed, enables the practitioner of tai chi chuan to move the body optimally and without effort. There is a structure to tai chi that you must put your body through to achieve the state of relaxation. After learning the sequence of movements, slow practice enables a person to be attentive to the body. Only by going slowly can you teach the body tai chi principles but, with time, your body will, e.g., 'tuck in' without being reminded. As the tuck becomes natural to your body, other principles can be programmed into the body, like 'roundness' and 'concave chest.' Gradually, with more practice and increased comfort with the sequence, it is possible for you to let your body tell *you* what to do. It will tell you where to position the hand and what is the correct movement of the leg.

Tai chi is a science. The tai chi principles are the natural laws of bodily movement. As you practice, you apply those laws and then observe and respond to the body's reaction. This feedback loop is how you progress toward the state of relaxation. You can only do this by doing the form slowly, and while doing the form slowly you constantly feel for your body's misalignment. When you feel a misalignment, you tell your body to adjust appropriately — fixing your alignment problems and healing yourself — in accordance with the tai chi principles. As mentioned above, eventually, you won't need to tell the body what to do; the body will tell you what to do. That is, you move the tai chi way: concaved, tucked-in, round, energy emanating from the *tan tien*, smooth, total integration of mind and body, and full development of 'you' as a human completely in tune with your environment.

## 2.25
## But how does relaxation come from the stress of following rules?

I used to teach physics. One experiment I did was hanging a string from the ceiling and tying a stone to the bottom of the string. If left alone, the stone will not move. It just hangs there. This means the tension of the string is very relaxed. But if you turn the stone in one direction, what happens? Inevitably, the stone will turn back in the other direction. The reason is because of the stress in the string. The stress will make the stone go back and forth until there is no more tension and the stone will stop moving.

Likewise, the body must find the least tension so that it is like the immobile stone hanging from the string in all it does. Take the Horse Stance, for instance: when you first assume the position you should feel like you can hold that posture for an indefinite amount of time. Why? You are relaxed because you are holding it correctly. As time goes by, while you are holding the stance, certain parts of the body will become uncomfortable. This means the body is sensing the weakest link of the chain and it is a positive sign for it means the body is fixing itself — healing itself. You cannot fix the body in one day: it takes time. Work on the Horse Stance every day and the benefits will accumulate. Like the string example, as the body fixes itself, the weak links will disappear and the stance can be held longer and longer with consistent practice over months and years.

The same principles apply to the tai chi form. If you have unnecessary stress while you do the form, the body will tell you it is incorrect. The best way to move the body is through relaxation and letting the mind guide the movement. If you are not relaxed, you cannot move properly. That's why we do it relaxed. If you do it tense, you miss the signal and intellectualize the whole thing. This is a mistake. Real tai chi is when the body tells you what to do. That's why I recommend you sometimes do the form when tired, so the body has no choice but to move correctly and not intellectually. There is so much the body can tell you. There are many layers of knowledge in doing slow tai chi. This is one of the interesting ones.

Remember, if you do tai chi wrong the body will tell you. The knee hurts. The back hurts. If you do it right, the knee and back get stronger. Alignment, relaxation and practicing slowly, may sound simple, yet they are crucial for learning.

## 2.26
## Is there a benefit similar to meditation from doing the form slow?

Slow tai chi heals the body as well as the mind. The process of learning the form, as described above, helps the mind too. At first, the mind concentrates on making the body do certain things — thus the mind is not worrying about daily life. Gradually, as the body relaxes and moves more correctly, the mind has also been trained to focus on the form. At this point, you can apply techniques from meditation: focusing on breathing as well as the meaning of the move.

## 2.27
## If tai chi is a martial art, why do the form slowly? How does that prepare a person to fight? Fights, after all, happen fast.

If you can do the form slowly and correctly, it means that you have the correct alignment, which is important in fighting.

Only by doing the tai chi form slowly can you find your 'curve' and become relaxed. As previously mentioned, doing the form slowly improves your alignment, which is discussed elsewhere. Part of developing the alignment is to find the proper position of your arm, for example, in a strike. Brush Knee can be a very effective strike in a fight but only if you have discovered the best curvature of your arm. The best curve will most effectively line up the body from palm to foot. Without that alignment the strike will be ineffective: one learns that alignment only by practicing slow, letting the body tell you the best position for it to be in for that move. Once the body learns the correct alignment, it will become second nature and you will not have to think about it when you need to use it. On the other hand, hurrying the body through the form leads to tension and weak alignment.

Secondly, relaxation makes the good fighter; a fighter who is not relaxed is not a good fighter. If you do the form correctly, slowly, and relaxed, the movements become second nature to you, meaning they become just they way you move. Relaxed does not mean limp, rather, it means your body is aligned correctly mentally and physically so that the moves occur without effort. Having trained your body to move correctly in this way, you will then be able to do the tai chi movements very fast. Moreover, in a fighting situation your body will respond automatically (without having to think or tense up) with those correct moves you trained the body to do. So, whoever trains to this level will stay relaxed all the time and if faced with a fight, he or she will 'let it be' — let the body do what it knows to do.

# III. TAI CHI & SELF-DEFENSE

## 3.1
### Is tai chi just for good health?

From the beginning, tai chi was practiced as a martial art. You can clearly see this in the classics by the old tai chi masters. It's important for a student to remember that tai chi is a fighting art. It is about striking, yielding, *nei kung* power, and such. All these elements should be emphasized when one studies the art. The tai chi classics and masters like Yang Cheng-fu, Wu Yu-hsiang, and Wu Chien-chuan talk about tai chi only as a martial art and never really detailed its health benefits or its relationship, if any, to meridian theory. Their writings spoke mainly about applications. A person who can apply tai chi to fighting must be agile and flexible enough to carry out the moves. So, tai chi is a fighting art that depends on having a healthy body and mind.

    Tai chi is not a New Age dance nor is it just an exercise. Tai chi is a way of life. When you practice tai chi correctly, good health follows as a matter of course. Good health is a prerequisite of being a good fighter and tai chi trains the whole body to work at its maximum in terms of striking power and in terms of the immune system's functioning. Whoever takes it up merely as a health exercise will miss the true intricacy and beauty of the art. The level of understanding of such a practitioner will be watered down as will the benefits derived.

## 3.2
### Do we get the same benefits learning tai chi for health as we do when learning it for self-defense?

You will get more benefit learning tai chi as self-defense than just for health. First of all, tai chi is a martial art — an art of fighting. So when you do tai chi you should think of it as a fighting art.

    To be a good fighter you must have a healthy body and mind. For example, you need to be strong to execute your attacking power. You also need good health in order to be rooted, agile, able to move back and forth swiftly and able to snap back at an opponent like a rubber band for counter offense. Doing tai chi for self-defense will give you good health as a matter of course.

### 3.3
### Am I missing something if I don't learn tai chi as self-defense?

The problem with people learning tai chi without learning the meaning and application of each move is that they will only get some of the benefits tai chi provides. In fact, without learning tai chi as a martial art, you'd be lucky to get the form 10% correct and get 10% of the possible health benefits.

Learning tai chi only for health is not enough for you to assess how correct your movements are. However, if you learn tai chi with self-defense in mind, you develop a feeling for the movements. For example, Brush Knee and Twist Step is a palm attack. If you just learn tai chi for health, you'll have no idea how to place the hand or what the hand should look like. You won't know if the palm should be higher or lower, or if the fingers should be bent. You just won't know the difference.

Brush Knee and Twist Step includes a yield and a strike; to do it, the body must be aligned correctly and the mind must be concentrating on the correct area. Power in tai chi comes from within: it is called *'i'* power (pronounced "yi") and comes from the mind. This is opposed to *'li'* which comes from localized muscle strength. Mind power, *i,* is developed over time by focusing the mind on the strike as the body lines up correctly for that strike. Tai chi relies on the mind concentrating on a strike composed of a correctly aligned body, and this integration of body and mind makes tai chi an effective fighting art as well as beneficial exercise. (For more on power see question 4.24 and *TCCP&P,* p. 8).

Only by learning tai chi as an art of self-defense (for example, ultimately practicing Brush Knee and Twist Step against a heavy bag or a partner with appropriate protection), can you get the most benefit out of the form. Knowing the meaning of the move and how to stick to an opponent and how to attack is the key to maximizing the benefit of the art. When you do any move in the form, the body needs to be lined up correctly and be rooted. The move needs to be linked to the rest of your body. It is important to understand that tai chi is objective and scientific. It is not subjective. There is a right way to do each move: a right way to hold the fist; a right way to hold the body; and a right way to move the body.

### 3.4
### But what if I am not interested in learning self-defense?

People say they don't want to learn self-defense because they see so much violence and the hurting of other people in the world generally and they don't want any part of it. But people need to be more realistic. Learning how to take care of yourself in any situation is very important. Often, the knowledge of self-defense and the philosophy of self-defense are essential. As the saying goes, "don't bury your head in the sand." At some point in time, self-defense may be necessary. It is intrinsic to all animals to know how to defend themselves in order to survive. Humans are no different. People should not ignore the body. In addition, knowing and practicing self-defense makes the body and mind strong and in harmony. All of these things take a long time.

There is a saying in China, "When the poet meets the tiger, no matter how many poems he recites, the tiger is not going to go away." Sometimes you must use self-defense. In today's society you will not meet a tiger, but you may meet a mugger or some crazy person who wants to hurt you or the people you love. If that happens, you can't be reciting poetry! You need to know some survival skills. You need to know some self-defense the same way you need to know how to drive a car or catch a fish or start a fire. It's good to know more about life than just your immediate environment and not be myopic.

Learning self-defense and becoming a "fighter" are two different things. Fighters are often trained athletes who compete against others as in a tournament. Self-defense is something we all need some basic knowledge of for self-preservation.

### 3.5
### Why should one engage in a practice aimed at hurting others?

The mechanism of self-defense is intrinsic to all animals. Human beings are animals too, just with more brainpower. When an animal moves in self-defense or for any other purpose, its entire body operates as one integral unit. In modern human societies, however, people seldom use such basic animal abilities such as running, jumping, climbing, or fighting in self-defense. But self-defense and the survival instinct are inherent in all species.

Let me emphasize that self-defense is not all about offense. Of course, the attacking moves are offensive; and sometimes we need to strike to immobilize the opponent temporarily. Tai chi can be a deadly effective martial art. However, tai chi is not primarily an art of offense. It is a system of defense emphasizing the principle of responding to the opponent and the situation. The statement "four ounces can deflect a thousand pounds" sums it up. With tai chi, an opponent or a difficult situation can be overcome by yielding to and redirecting the force that comes at us.

Over time people realized that tai chi was good for health too. It has become one of the most popular health exercises practiced today. At my school, tai chi is taught as a martial art and the health benefits are considered bonuses. In his book *The Art of War,* Sun Tzu says, "the best general wins a battle without fighting; the second best one wins it by fighting." Likewise, the aim of tai chi is to win without fighting or with the least amount of force. Fighting is the last resort. A high-level tai chi practitioner would not need to engage in a struggle to overcome an opponent, whereas a low-level fighter would have to rely mostly on external and localized strength to stop the opponent. They say a cornered dog will bite. One should learn enough fighting skills so as not to become cornered.

The person who trains in tai chi seriously will have a better awareness and sensitivity. Therefore he or she will avoid or neutralize many potential confrontations before they happen or get out of control. Push-hands teaches the body to yield, but the concept of yielding begins with a calm yet alert mind. As I often say, yielding is not losing. Yielding is repositioning as in a game of chess.

### 3.6
### What makes tai chi unique and effective as a system of self-defense?

I would say that there are four elements that make tai chi unique as a system of self-defense: yielding, internal power, rootedness and body integration.

### 3.7
### What is "yielding" in tai chi?

There is a story told about a tai chi master (attributed to Yang Jianhou, Yang Cheng-fu's father) whose ability to yield was developed to such a high degree that a bird standing on his palm would not be able to fly away. When a bird flies, it must initially push its feet against something and then flap its wings. When the bird tried to push off, the master would withdraw his hand just enough so that the bird could not find any resistance to push against. Without resistance from the master's palm, the bird was unable to fly away. This illustrates Newton's third law of motion, which says, "for every action there is an equal and opposite reaction." If the hand offers resistance, the bird can push down (action) and fly away (reaction). Without resistance, there can be no reaction. Likewise, to yield is to bend to the opponent so that his strike doesn't find resistance, something to push against.

When an attacking strike occurs, if the target moves (thus offering no resistance), then there is no strike (the strike is not completed). Or rather, the strike just misses. If the target of the strike follows the hit, allowing it to spend itself, then the target is yielding. To yield is to remove the reaction from the attack's action. By moving aside and sticking to the attacking arm, the object has moved but not in reaction to the strike, so the striking force is canceled. By yielding, there is nothing to push against (as with the bird above). Another way to explain it is, at a high level, tai chi fighters let people touch them but give them nothing to strike. As above, the bird touches the hand but can find no resistance to push against. Another commonly used figure of speech to explain this concept follows: when facing an opponent, be like cotton; he can sense the cotton is there but he can find nothing to hit. If you offer no resistance, the opponent has nothing to hit.

The concept of yielding is summed up by the classic tai chi expression, "use four ounces of power to deflect the force of a thousand pounds." Essentially, this means that a tai chi practitioner should not resist an opponent's attacking force. Instead, he should yield, using a minimum amount of force to deflect the opponent's attack. Then, he can make an effective counterattack.

A high-level tai chi practitioner stays as close to his opponent as a matador stays to a charging bull. When the time is appropriate, he counter-strikes perpendicular to the attacking force. In certain retreating moves, the defender coils backwards to yield, as if compressing a spring, and creating significant potential energy. If the defender is properly positioned and rooted, even a relatively limited amount of his potential energy can have a great effect on a strong, fast-moving opponent. Yielding is repositioning. Yielding is not losing. It's like a game of chess: you reposition yourself, and each move is to gain advantage.

### 3.8
### What is internal power?

Internal power is *nei kung*, which is a series of exercises that strengthens the body and circulates the *chi*. *Nei kung* increases the density and flexibility of the bones, strengthens the internal organs and systems (immune, circulatory, etc.), and, most importantly, it makes the muscles and fascia wrapping around the body strong. Think of the difference between a young tree and an old tree. The old tree is brittle. The young tree is strong and elastic. That is what *nei kung* and internal power is about. (For more information see *The Book of Nei Kung* and chapter 6.)

### 3.9
### You mentioned rootedness in self-defense. What exactly is it?

A fifty-pound log that is just lying on the ground can be moved easily. However, a live tree weighing fifty pounds is much more difficult to move because it is rooted to the earth. When a tai chi practitioner delivers an attack, he positions himself as if his whole body's mass were linked to the ground like a tree.

How does the tai chi practitioner achieve rooting? By adjusting his body alignment in such a way as to increase the friction between his body and the floor during each attacking or yielding movement. This is one of the fundamental principles in *nei kung*, and one of the reasons *nei kung* is so important to proper practice of tai chi.

Most other fighting systems depend heavily on speed and localized muscular strength. While speed and strength are important, there are limits to how much one can increase them. On the other hand, rootedness and internal power can be increased almost infinitely. They are the most important factors in self-defense skills in tai chi. With internal power, one can deliver stronger attacks as well as take punishment without injury. With rootedness, one becomes "immovable" as if stuck to the ground, so the opponent feels as if he's slamming into a solid wall.

### 3.10
### What is full-body integration?

Another important element is what I call full-body integration. Here, all parts of the body work as one unit. With a punch, the movement of the hand is fully connected with the rest of the body. Breath, *chi* movement and mind power are also integrated and must move together during the punch. This means that the mind, the breath, the root, the twist, and the speed of the punch are completely unified. Integration of the body also allows us to use our own strength more efficiently. The hand connects to an opponent during a strike; but obviously the hand that moves by itself from the wrist does not have much strength. When the back, torso, waist, and legs are linked into one mass behind the movement of that hand, and that mass is rooted, the strength of integration can be realized (for more see *TCCP&P,* p. 18).

### 3.11
### Is too much yielding bad or unbalanced?

There is no such thing as too much yielding. Yielding is responding to an opponent's attack. You do this by staying close to the opponent as he attacks, so that he can touch you but not move you. You remain balanced while moving, able to get away from any attack and still control the situation. How much you yield depends entirely on the attack — small attack, small yield. As in the game of chess, the aim of fighting is to checkmate the opponent. You use yielding to position or align yourself behind the opponent's power in order to be in control. Roll Back is a good example of how to control an opponent's hand and elbow. It puts him in an awkward position and off-balance, so he cannot counterattack. It is like a checkmate: the game is over. This is correct yielding. Incorrect yielding, however, means staying too far away from the opponent and not close enough to checkmate him. Students learn the distinction by practicing push-hands.

### 3.12
### Tai Chi has an image that is very different from what most people associate with "martial arts."

Hard-style martial arts have a reputation for violence and aggression, because many of their students feel the need to show how tough they are, or demonstrate how much injury they are capable of causing. Often these schools emphasize attacking skills, or dramatic stunts like breaking boards.

Hurting people is not difficult with a little bit of martial arts training. The tai chi approach — neutralizing the opponent's force (with push-hands training) and absorbing his punch (*nei kung* training) while maintaining control of the situation — is extremely difficult. One can always find a way to hurt others in a tit-for-tat test of toughness, but that is not an art. Developing the skills, sensitivity, and openness to respond to whatever comes your way is the art of tai chi.

Within the martial arts world there is criticism that tai chi takes too long to learn. However, no reputable master of any style will deny that the soft, internal style characteristic of tai chi is the highest level of martial art.

### 3.13
### Other martial arts seem easier and faster to learn.

Obviously, less complex fighting systems are easier to learn. For example, some schools let a student fight in the very first class. While it is fine to move around and get a little exercise, what can anyone really know about fighting at that stage, and what can that student be capable of learning in the first periods of training? To make a one-story building does not require a substantial foundation. But if the aspiration is to build a skyscraper, then the first act must be to dig downward. In tai chi, a student must dig down and build a strong foundation. That is why tai chi begins with slow movements. Building up comes later, say, by developing speed.

### 3.14
### What makes martial art fighting different from a bar fight?

Fighting is fighting, whether or not one uses kung fu. The difference is the motive behind the fighting. Bar fighters beat each other up simply to "teach a lesson," but not to destroy or kill. Of course, accidents can happen and someone can get seriously injured or killed, but that's the not the intention. Their brawls are shows of strength, and anything goes. Martial arts, on the other hand, were created specifically for combat on battlefields and therefore are more deadly.

### 3.15
### If tai chi is a fighting art, why are some of its movements so flowing and aesthetically pleasing to the eye? Combat, more often than not, is brutal and chaotic. Explain the paradox.

The tai chi form is a fixed sequence of movements. Prior to choreographing the postures into the traditional form sequence, postures were practiced one at a time. A fighter would do the posture over and over again, oftentimes opposite a partner doing an appropriate responding posture. Eventually, the postures were linked together into one form as both a training device and a mnemonic device. Without this fixed sequence, tai chi would be lost to history. Each teacher may focus on certain techniques, but the sequence of movements is always there as a foundation never to be forgotten. Accordingly, the tai chi practitioner always knows what move should come next, whether the form is being done fast or slow. With the sequence as a foundation, the student can learn combat, application of the form in push-hands, *san shou*, and sparring. The person training to fight can break the form up (*san* means chopping up or not continuous, and *shou* means hand) and drill individual movements against a partner or a bag to build power in those moves. That is why my students learn *san shou* in Fighting Class after they become proficient in the form. In Fighting Class students drill individual moves. To drill a move is, for example, to do Grasp Bird's

Tail (Left) repeatedly in order to train the body to do the move correctly. The tai chi form sequence is only the foundation.

Through practice and the help of a teacher, the execution of the form should be aesthetically pleasing. If it is not, it suggests that the practitioner has some kind of physical problem — maybe a weak hip — that needs to be fixed. In fighting, of course, there is no set sequence to follow and no way of predicting what will happen. Instead, tai chi teaches you to respond to an opponent's unpredictable changes. After a move, whether attacking or yielding, you must reorient to respond to the next situation in the best way. Knowing how to execute tai chi moves correctly, you can always maintain balance despite the unpredictability. The series of such spontaneous moves may look chaotic to an untrained eye. However, someone who understands tai chi can find them elegant as he sees clearly what the fighters are doing, and how they position themselves to yield or attack.

In a fight, the form is chopped up but those with a trained eye can see particular movements. For example, my students drill Heel Kick and Side Kick both right and left nearly every week. Drills are for training and the movements should be done correctly while drilling so the body develops the ability to execute that particular strike. So, in the drills, the student should do a Heel Kick correctly and with beauty, lifting the hands and elbows a certain way. But if a situation in real life arises calling for a Heel Kick — just kick, don't worry about the elbows. So tai chi is a system that trains the whole body so that when the opportunity arises, the right movement will be used naturally and with necessary efficiency.

Tai chi training follows certain principles because that is the proven method for developing fighting ability. Someone who does tai chi correctly moves like a motor that spins very fast. His moves look nice, smooth and quiet. However, when that seemingly elegant punch or kick is applied in fighting, it will have a brutal impact on the opponent.

Actually, a good fighter, when applying tai chi in a fight, should look elegant too. You can see the fighter yield, tuck and be round. For example, a high kick can be done beautifully, but if that high kick connects to someone you see the brutal hit. A race car accelerates from zero to sixty miles an hour in three seconds and you will see the elegance of the car maneuvering, but if this car hits something it will be brutal. The same thing is true of a punch. A punch can be real fast and elegant, but if it hits something it's brutal, yet still elegant. However, most people just see the result and don't have a trained eye to see the elegance of the attack.

### 3.16
### People have such different types of energy. While yielding, I feel like I am losing myself — I become a chameleon, adapting to each person. How do I yield but also maintain my own goal and energy?

It is correct practice to adapt to one's partner. It is just like a social dance in which the female dancer must follow the lead of her partner. The male partner is active (*yang*) while the female partner is passive (*yin*). However, that is only the yielding part of practice. In fighting, yielding to let the opponent lead, as it were, is also a search for an opportunity to counterattack. If you just let him lead or get lost in his lead, then you are led — simple as that — and he has his way with you. Instead, tai chi teaches that when it is the right time, reposition and use attacking techniques to overcome him. When is the right time? Well, you should be looking for it; if the attack is from the front, step to the side and counterattack perpendicularly to the strike. The first thing one must learn in push-hands is yielding and it is an excellent technique to have. However, the practice is not complete without learning the attacking techniques of how to tip the opponent being yielded to off balance. In self-defense, the combination of skills in push-hands and fighting are both equally essential. Yielding forever is not the answer; attack at some point and overcome the opponent.

### 3.17
### How can we learn how to fight if we practice in "slow-motion"?

Someone was quoted in *T'ai Chi Magazine* as saying that tai chi can only be used successfully in self-defense against a slow-motion mugger. That person, who is actually a tai chi teacher, has missed the whole point. He doesn't understand tai chi at all. Eventually, tai chi moves should be done as fast as possible. When these moves are applied in self-defense, they obviously need to be executed quickly. Most people only see a slow, meditative form of tai chi often being practiced by elderly people. Those who see only the slow form don't know that a fast practice exists.

To learn something properly, whether it is to be done quickly or slowly, one should be calm and relaxed. Consider a figure skating or gymnastics routine. Those athletes do not do those moves fast their first day. The same goes for tai chi. Nobody can learn the moves and do them fast right away. It takes time for the body to learn how to move correctly to execute the moves.

Tai chi principles of movement are easy to recite: head suspended, knees over toes, lower back straight (tucked-in), the whole body rounded and rooted, breathing slow and deep, coordinating breath and movement, and so on. Once recited, they remain difficult to master and coordinate, even in slow motion. Maintaining balance, for example, is more challenging when moving slowly. To experience this, try to execute a high front kick or sidekick slowly, and see how difficult it is. So the student should always practice slowly. However, after becoming somewhat familiar with the movements, begin to practice them at the speed of actual fighting applications. Eventually, provided the movements are executed correctly, the faster the better.

### 3.18
### Is it true that no matter how slow our pace is, we should always work at going slower?

Yes, but also work at being faster for fighting applications. Once comfortable working with the tai chi principles in a slow practice, try to push both ends of the spectrum.

True, it is more fundamental to slow down. That is where coordination comes from. As the tai chi classics say, "extreme softness can later become extreme hardness," which is to say, "fastness comes from slowness" (*TCCP&P*, p. 81). This means that we must ultimately face fast movement as part of our work in tai chi.

### 3.19
### Does tai chi develop confidence in fighting?

Certainly, by knowing how to yield the tai chi way, through the practice of push-hands, gaining balance and control of any situation is a matter of course. Through tai chi training you gain confidence first, by learning how to get away due to the study of yielding. For the most part, the best response to an unavoidable confrontation is to get away. Next, with *nei kung* training, the body becomes strong enough to withstand the impact of hard attacks. Thus, with yielding and a strong body, a tai chi practitioner has a real confidence and a solid capacity to handle situations. In other martial arts they train to have guts and to tough it out; in tai chi, we train to have confidence.

There's an old saying: "If a dog comes toward you and you think it's a wolf, it will attack." This means that if we approach a dog defensively, it will respond by attacking. Similarly, sit next to a friendly person and assume he's aggressive, and you invite discord. Tai chi develops calmness so that the friendly dogs can be distinguished from the wolves. Thus, unnecessary aggression won't be stirred up or provoked. Tai chi gives us calmness, responsiveness, confidence and fighting skills.

### 3.20
### Is tai chi self-defense suitable for women?

Absolutely. Suppose a one-hundred-pound woman, standing five-foot-three, were to encounter a six-foot-tall, two-hundred-pound man. As a student of tai chi, she would learn to take advantage of her smaller size and weight by moving faster than her heavier opponent — much like a sports car outmaneuvering a truck. She would learn how to yield. One of the first principles of tai chi is yielding. So when the punch comes in she can move with the punch. In fact, at a high level she can even let the person's attack touch her, but she can stick to the attack and go behind the power and strike. Of course, that is not easy to learn; it takes many years of training.

On the other hand, if she had been training for many years in a hard-style school, she would have a hard time dealing with her opponent. This is because such systems emphasize blocking or using force against force. But it is simple physics: she can never exert more force than he can. In comparison, tai chi would help her develop rootedness and internal power so that she would be able to deliver power with greater speed and coordination than a heavier opponent. In fact, when at a disadvantage with height and/or weight no one should attempt to block or use force against force. This is again like the car/truck example, for although a sports car can outmaneuver a truck, it cannot survive a head-on collision with one.

As discussed above, as a student of tai chi develops rootedness, body mass effectively increases. As a result, her ability to yield and counterattack also increases. Additionally, with *nei kung* (or "iron vest" training), her body will be better able to sustain a strong blow. Finally, a woman should particularly appreciate the unique psychology of tai chi. Hard-style thinking sells women the idea that they can, or must be, just as tough as a man or tougher. The basic principle intrinsic to tai chi is that whether you are male or female, tall or short, young or old, you have certain strengths that can be utilized. Part of tai chi training is learning to recognize those attributes and to use them. As a matter of fact, all the attributes of tai chi serve to overcome a stronger opponent or more than one opponent.

### 3.21
### In addition to using the attributes of tai chi to overcome a stronger opponent, can they be used against more than one opponent?

In the old days, it was not uncommon for one person to fight a dozen or more people. It is hard to imagine, but they could handle weapons and swords and would move fast but not be out of breath.

This can be only partly experienced today. No matter how big a person is — 200 or 300 pounds — if they don't apply their body correctly, they are very clumsy. Application of techniques learned in tai chi class in everyday life results in advantages of grace and balance. Also, everyone has advantages or disadvantages; you need only to recognize them. For example, a tall person has long reach, so a short person must train something else. Remember that any attribute, such as localized muscular strength or height, can be an advantage under certain circumstances but a hindrance in others. Through tai chi training, the differences can be recognized and developed.

### 3.22
### Is tai chi fighting something I can pick up quickly?

No. You should learn it step by step and that takes time. Learning to be a fighter in the tai chi system is not easy. There are many more skills to learn than in other systems because to do it elegantly requires conditioning the body both physically and mentally. Physically, the body must be aligned correctly to execute the moves and breathing must be done correctly (long, deep, small, smooth). This physical training occurs while learning the slow form (as well as *chi kung* and *nei kung*), progressing to the fast form, then the slow and fast long form, as well as developing proficiency in push-hands before learning combat. Some systems let you fight the first day. In tai chi, fighting doesn't occur until after two years of training, at least. Skill in the tai chi system takes years to achieve.

I can't see how anyone will get all these things correct when treating tai chi as just some exercise. Just because in the beginning movement is slow and dance-like, does not mean it is a dance. Doing the form slow teaches balance, coordination, alignment, yielding, striking, and harmony of the mind and body. We do it slowly so that we can actually feel and know that every part of the body is integrated together, and moving correctly.

Doing tai chi slowly is not easy. For example, it is very difficult to execute a slow high kick. Once it can be done slowly, then it should be done faster and faster. Also, the power of the kick is based on whether you are tucking in and rooted and whether the whole body is connected in one piece.

### 3.23
### How many years of practice are required before one can successfully apply tai chi fighting techniques in the outside world?

That depends on several factors: how many hours one practices at home, the level of one's natural athletic ability, and, most importantly, what kinds of conditions exist if and when self-defense is needed. In general, it takes about half a year to learn the tai chi short form. Then, a student can begin learning push-hands and fighting. It will take about a year of practice to become familiar with the basic fighting techniques, although obviously much more time and effort is required to develop mastery. It is possible that within about two years of consistent practice, a student can develop the fundamental skills required for basic self-defense.

### 3.24
### Why is the palm used more than the fist in tai chi?

A palm strike is natural because the palm is a very strong part of the body. In evolutionary terms, humans used to walk on all fours and the palm is strong in the same way as a foot that stomps on things is strong. On the other hand, the fist is unnatural. Successful use of fist strikes requires training the hand, the knuckles, and the wrist as one integrated unit.

For example, you need to work on the alignment of the hand holding the fist. You need to know whether you are using the first two knuckles or the last two knuckles when connecting the punch. This uses a different kind of strength and needs to be trained to become strong. But the palm is naturally strong.

Another advantage of using the palm is that it is an open hand ready for another technique if needed. It can grab, hook, whip, and so on. This is why there are not too many fist strikes in tai chi. This is one of the many ways tai chi differs from other styles of kung fu.

### 3.25
### How do you make your palm stronger, how do you train your fist?

The palm is easy to use because it is naturally intrinsic to the body. To train the palm is called 'iron palm training.' This type of training is often depicted in kung fu movies in a sequence showing the hero training for combat. Training involves hitting the relaxed, open palm against something hard many times over a long period of time. (Consult a teacher or experienced trainer who has done this before doing it yourself.) At the beginning, the palm strikes a bag of beans, say. Gradually, the object becomes harder: a sand bag, then a bag of gravel, then of pebbles, then solid wood, then maybe stone, and then iron. It takes a few years, obviously, to train through all these steps. To accelerate training, a special lineament is applied to speed healing. The purpose of this training is to increase the density of the hand without diminishing any of its sensitivity. Do it incorrectly and the hand becomes an insensitive club. A similar process can be followed for developing the fist (that is, strike a succession of harder objects with the bare fist over a period of time). You can also strengthen the fingers by jabbing them into bowls of successively harder objects (like you see in movies).

If you have ever noticed how your feet change if you go for a long time barefoot, then you understand what this type of training is all about. By wearing shoes all the time, the feet grow soft and weak. But going barefoot for a long time, the feet become increasingly dense. Some people can play soccer or run marathons in bare feet because they have spent perhaps their whole life not wearing shoes. Same idea for 'iron palm training,' where you hit your hands against something hard over a period of time and the density of the hand will increase. Nowadays, nobody needs this type of training since hand-to-hand combat is not a daily affair. However, as I pointed out in 3.1 above, good health of the body and mind is intrinsic to high-level tai chi training.

### 3.26
### How does a relaxed fist that is trained correctly penetrate deeper than a stiff one?

First, *i,* mind power, is used to move the hand (see 3.3). A relaxed fist moves faster than a stiff one. In general, power is generated from the *tan tien* linked to the torso from the body's rootedness.

The proper delivery of a strike can be described in mathematical terms. The question is really how to put maximum energy behind a fist. A fist is an object in motion and its energy is kinetic energy. Kinetic energy is one half of the mass times the velocity squared ($E_k = \frac{1}{2}mv^2$). Very simply put, if the speed of the fist doubles, then the kinetic energy quadruples. The fist moves fastest when relaxed. Relaxation enables the body to align properly so that the torso, hips, and legs are all behind the fist. Finally, the alignment facilitates rootedness which increases the "striking power" of the mass geometrically, because a proper rootedness links your mass to the mass of the ground. A powerful fist is composed of (1) speed, (2) integrated body (see question 3.10 for more information), and (3) rootedness.

In general, stiffness is to be avoided in tai chi because power in tai chi originates as a wave in the *tan tien* which is expressed, like the end of a whip, in the fist or fingertips (see questions 5.6 & 5.15). Bulging, stiff muscles will inhibit the smoothness of the movement. Stiffness slows movement and leads to misalignment. For example, the weightlifter with bulging muscles can lift you up and choke you but he cannot throw a speedy, effective punch at you because he is muscle-bound. His muscles are not for striking, only for lifting weight. But to strike, you must train the whole body to align behind the punch. The power of an attack lies in the integration of the body parts.

### 3.27
### What are Silk Reeling and Spiral Power? Are The Compass, Rhino Gazes at the Moon, Owl Turns His Head and Cloud Hands (Stationary feet) examples of Silk-Reeling exercises?

The concepts of "silk reeling" and "spiral power" are analogous. They are simply two different ways of looking at how power is generated. The expressions may sound mysterious, but they are merely translations of Chinese terms. Silk reeling is a direct translation of a phrase used by old masters to explain to their students how the body moves.

In fighting, one must use the whole body as one instrument. The body always moves in somewhat circular movements. Therefore, even a simple straight punch is not delivered in a straight line. Here, silk reeling can be seen in the spiraling motion of the hand. A punch lacks power if there is no turning of the hand.

There are not many who can explain silk reeling, and many misunderstand it. All tai chi movements contain silk reeling in that everything twists and spirals. Correct movements utilize internal power (*nei kung*) and start from the *tan tien*. If one moves from the shoulders or the hips instead, little power is achieved. I would use the analogy of a running motor to explain power. A motor that spins fast is quiet, but it cannot spin fast if it wobbles. It is the same in tai chi. If the body wobbles and does not move from the *tan tien*, the power is limited. To learn to move correctly from the *tan tien*, one will need a teacher with a good understanding of the mechanism. If one does tai chi just for health and does not study the martial aspect, one will never understand this principle.

Indeed, the Compass and other moves mentioned above are silk reeling exercises. Cloud Hands may be the best example for most people. If I were to describe silk reeling, I would say, "it is power spiraling from the *tan tien* and it gives more power when delivering a fighting move."

### 3.28
### In fighting, do we ever set a trap to lure an opponent?

In general, don't try to set traps in tai chi. Traps are for war and for offense. A person or an army plans violence against an enemy and sets a trap for that purpose. Traps are used by those seeking violence, and that is not a principle of tai chi.

Tai chi trains you correctly for self-defense. The key to self-defense, the key idea of tai chi, is responding. Tai chi training prepares you to defend yourself from an attack from any direction and any side at any moment. High-level fighters are able to respond to any situation, so there is no need to worry about setting a trap.

Tournament competitions are the exception because of the imposed time constraints. You don't actually set up a trap, but you do have certain combinations that follow one another that you plan to use. Tai chi training is a training in response. This means that moves are combined (see *TCCP&P,* p. 23). A simple combination would be straight punch left, then right or a punch followed by a kick or front kick followed by a side kick. That latter combination assumes someone is in front of you and to the side of you. If you are thinking about setting a trap all the time, you are not thinking about responding. Combinations in tournament competitions are not really traps.

### 3.29
### When striking an opponent, what is the correct distance to place oneself for maximum power?

I call this focusing. It's like having an old-fashioned camera. You need to calculate in your head the distance of the object you are photographing. If the object is too far or too close, you're not in focus and the picture will be blurred.

Fighting is similar. Too far or close, your power is not maximized. You need to adjust your distance. Learning to adjust your distance requires many steps of training. These steps are taught in push-hands and fighting classes.

### 3.30
### Have you ever had to use self-defense in real life?

Many times. Growing up in Hong Kong there were fistfights all the time. Since leaving Hong Kong, it has happened twice. Both times I was involved in fighting more than a half a dozen opponents. One time I was in the street in Chinatown (NYC) and the other time I was in a restaurant bar in Taiwan. The latter incident was just like a kung fu movie, the tables were turned over — there was chaos. I just responded to the situation and as quickly as it began all the opponents disappeared. Both times, if I had not known self-defense I would have been seriously injured. Instead, I emerged without a scratch. As usual with such incidents, they happen when you least expect it but, when they do occur, it is good to have some knowledge of self-defense.

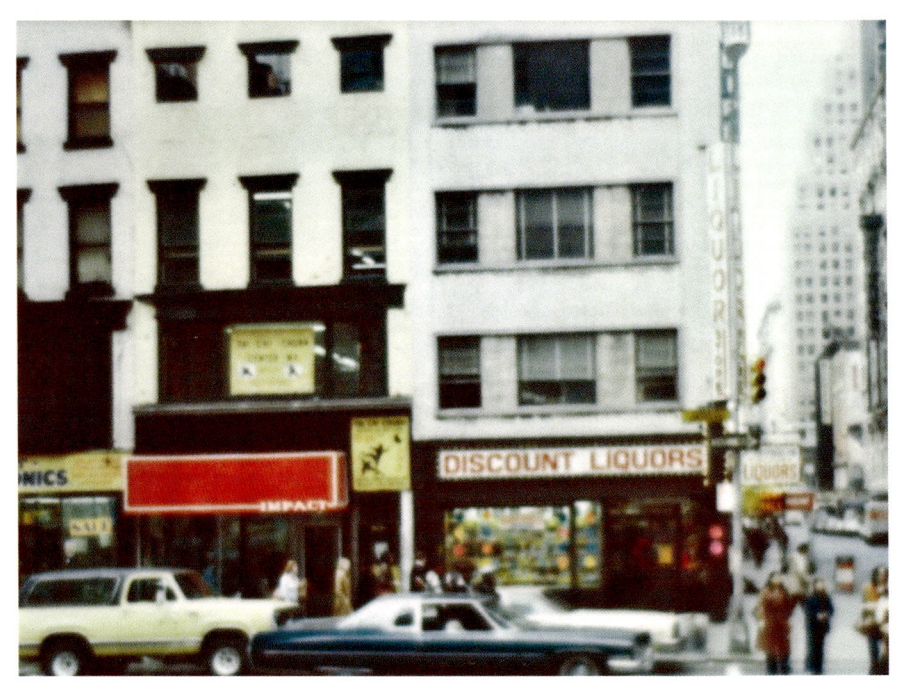

The first location of the Tai Chi Chuan Center were the second and third floors of 1117 Avenue of the Americas from 1973-1989.

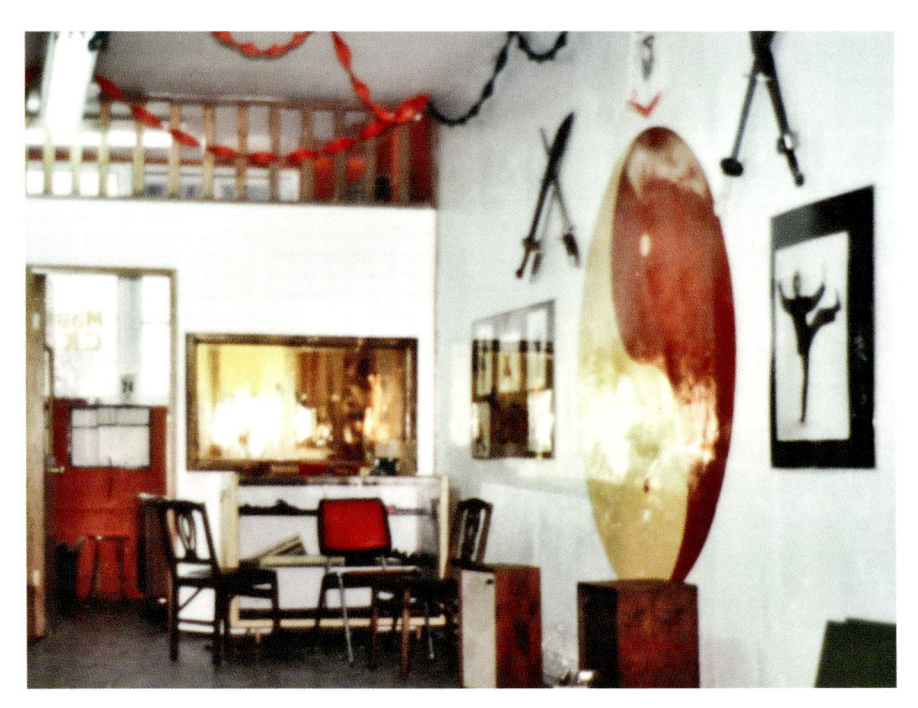

Inside the first Tai Chi Chuan Center.

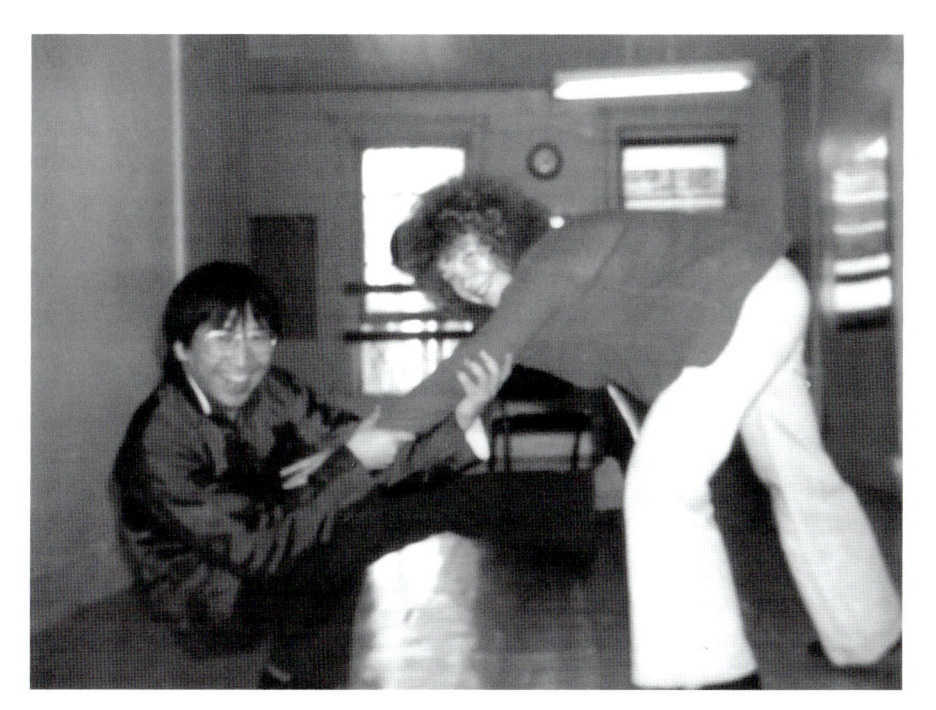

Master Chu, in the first school, demonstrating yielding all the way down during push-hands.

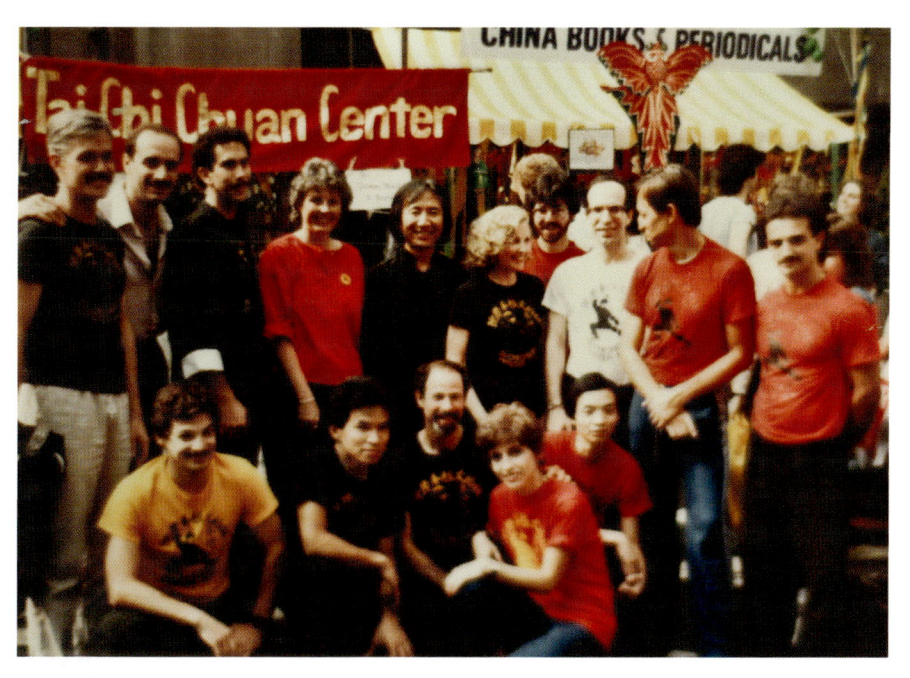

From the beginning, students of the Tai Chi Chuan Center educated the public about tai chi. This is a group photo of students who participated in the Fifth Avenue Book Fair in the 1980s. Peter Julian (top row, white shirt), Hing Ying Chu (bottom row, far right), and Ira Michael (bottom row, yellow shirt), were teaching assistants at the time.

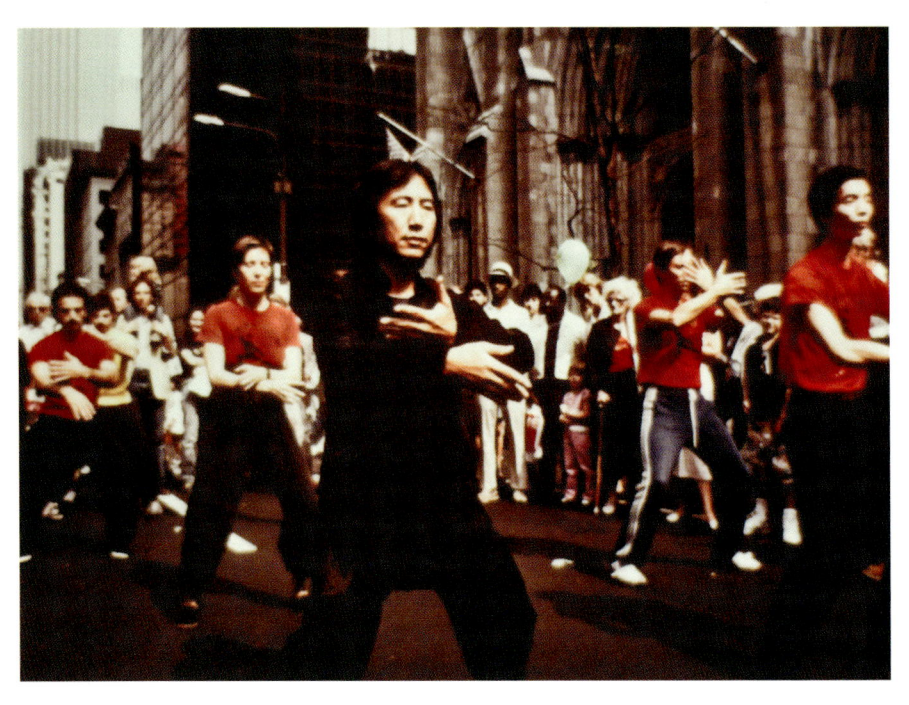

Master Chu leads a group of students in the tai chi form in front of St. Patrick's Cathedral as part of the Fifth Avenue Book Fair.

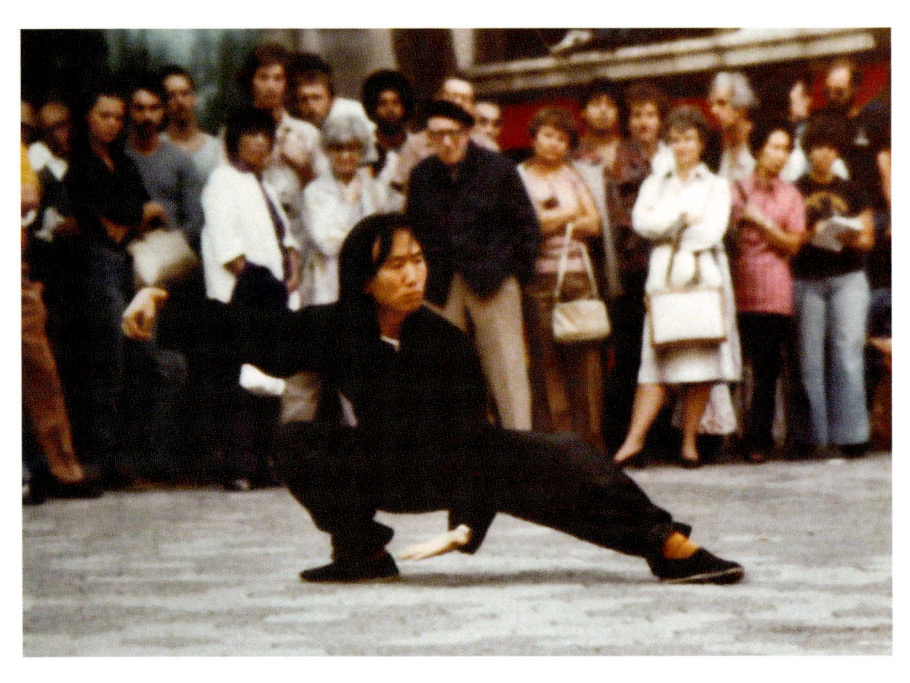

Master Chu demonstrating the tai chi form in Columbus Park, Chinatown (1978). In the background, Sophia Delza (see 1.14) is the one wearing a white jacket (fourth from left). From the beginning, Master Chu's school has been a force in the kung fu community.

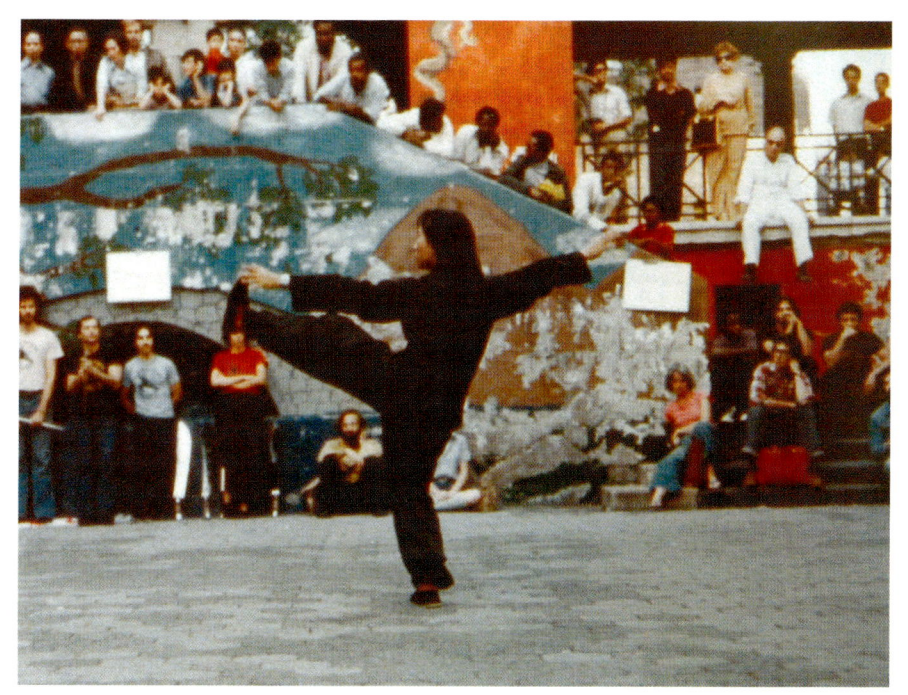

Master Chu demonstrating the tai chi form in Columbus Park.

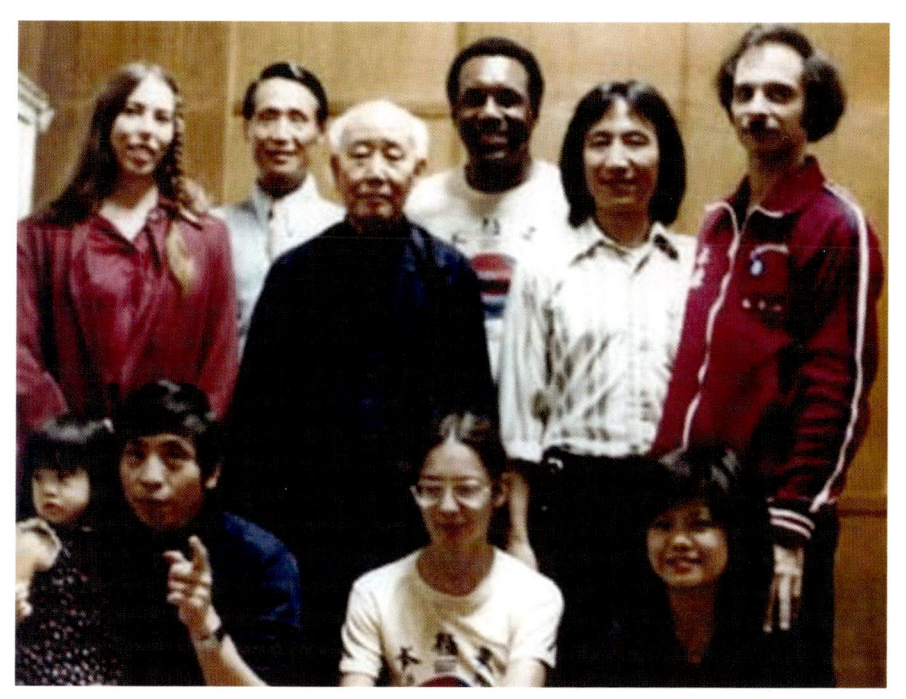

An assembly of tai chi masters in the 1970s: T.T. Liang is in the center. Crouching in the lower left is William C C Chen. First on the right is Frank de Maria, second from the right is C K Chu, third is Sidney Austin. Second from the left is Jou Tsung Hwa.

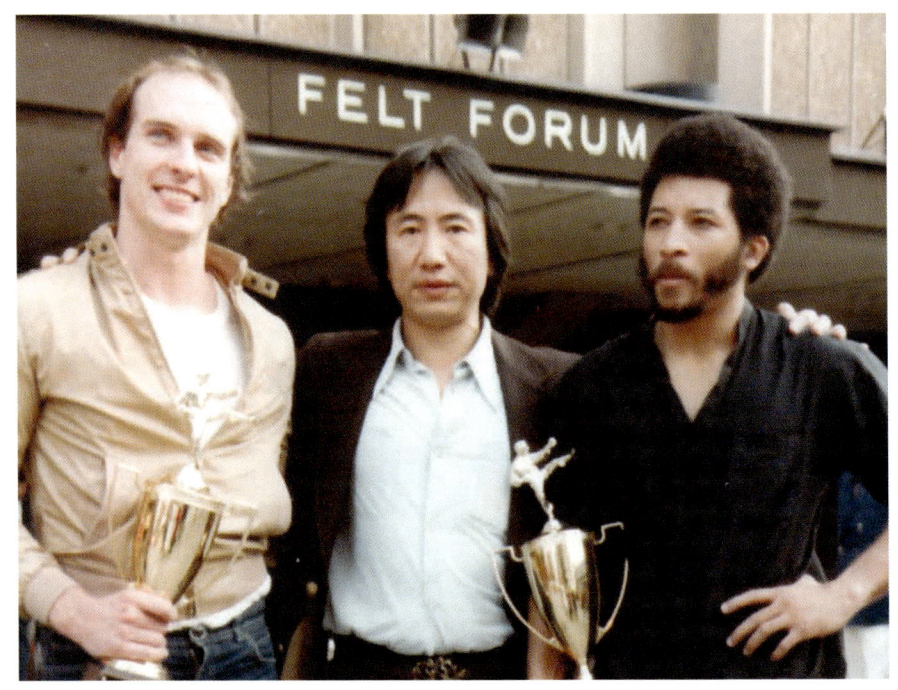

Vincent Sobers and Richard Trybulski of the Tai Chi Chuan Center captured Middleweight and Heavyweight titles by knockout at the first and last kung fu tournament in Madison Square Gardens.

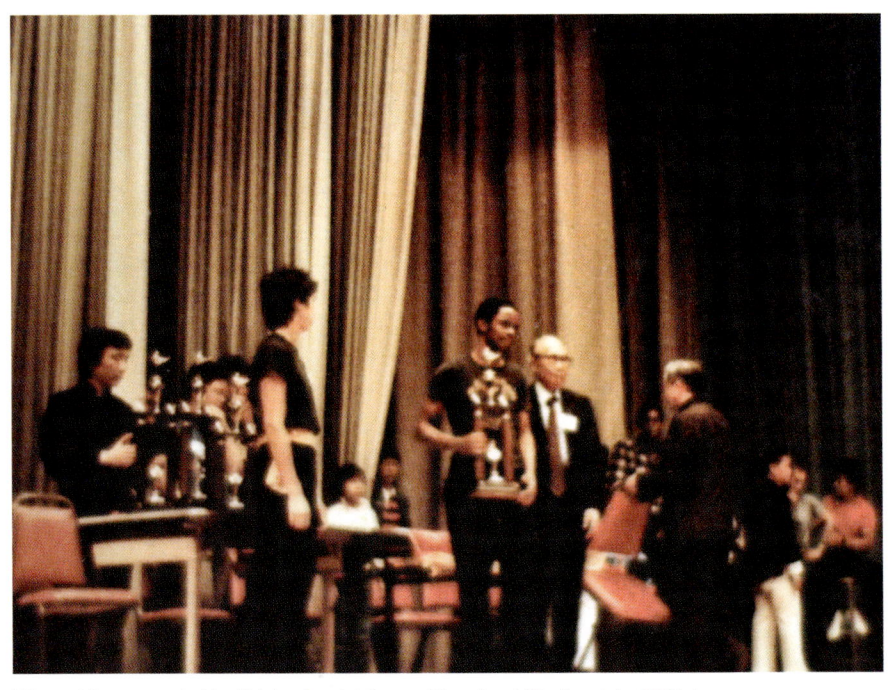

Edmund Berry won in his division by yielding and knockout (Boston, late 1970s).

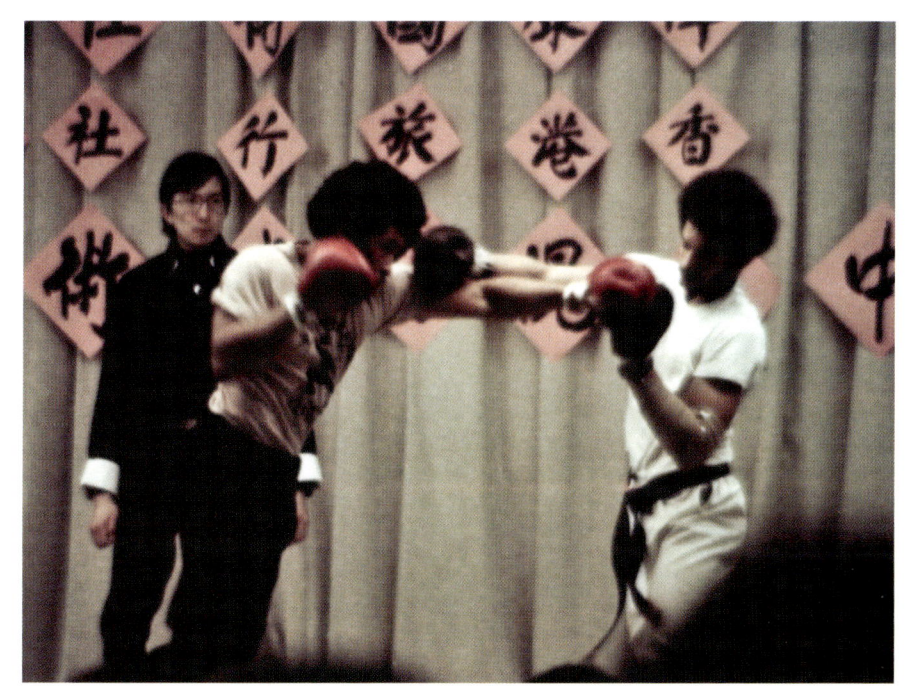

Vincent Sobers (on the left) in an elimination match (Boston, late 1970s).

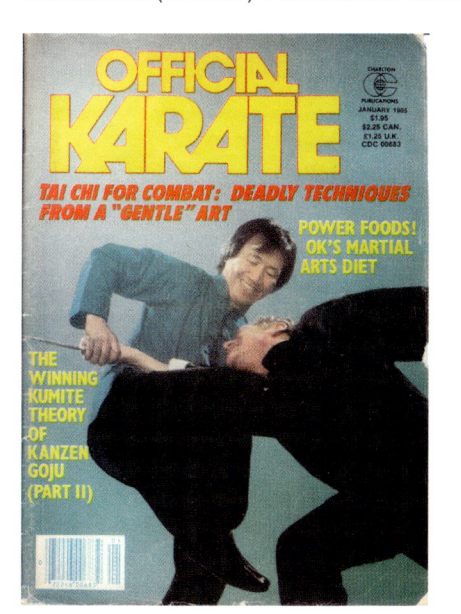

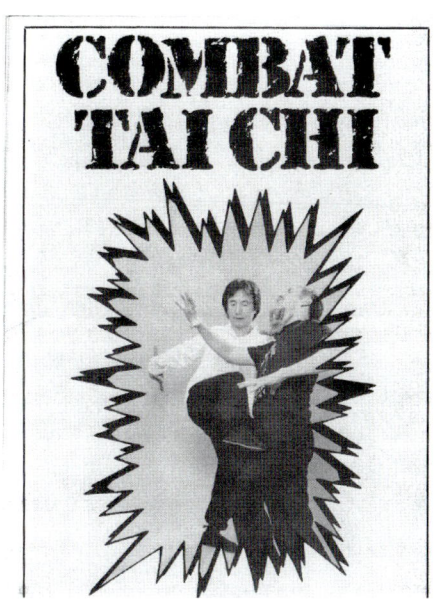

Master Chu has made many appearances on TV, including the Mike Douglas Show, and has been featured in many magazine articles, like *Official Karate* and *Inside Kung Fu*.

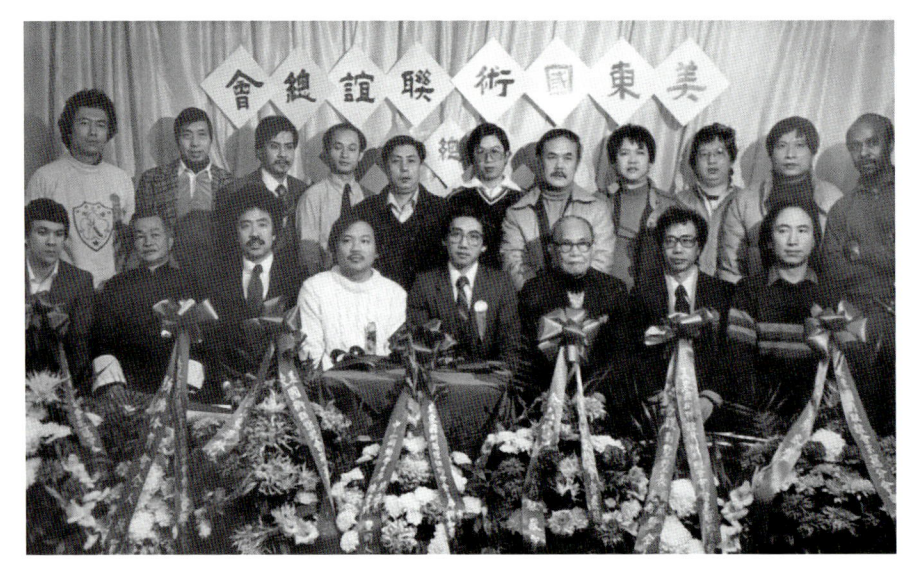

All Kung-fu Masters Exhibition 1983. *Front Row (from left)*: 1. Paul Vizzio, future Golden Gloves winner (Fu Jow Pai); 2. Kwang Tit-fu (Hung Gar); 4. Tony Lau (Hung Gar); 5. Fong Ji Yu (Fu Jow Pai); 8. C. K. Chu. *Back Row:* 1. Tony Chuy, Sifu's brother (Praying Mantis); 2. William C C Chen (Tai Chi); 4. Chan Ton Fai (White Crane); 5.Wan Chi Ming (Hung Gar); 7. Leung Shum (Eagle Claw); 9. Wing Hong Yip (Dragon Style); 10. Kenny Gong (Hsing-I).

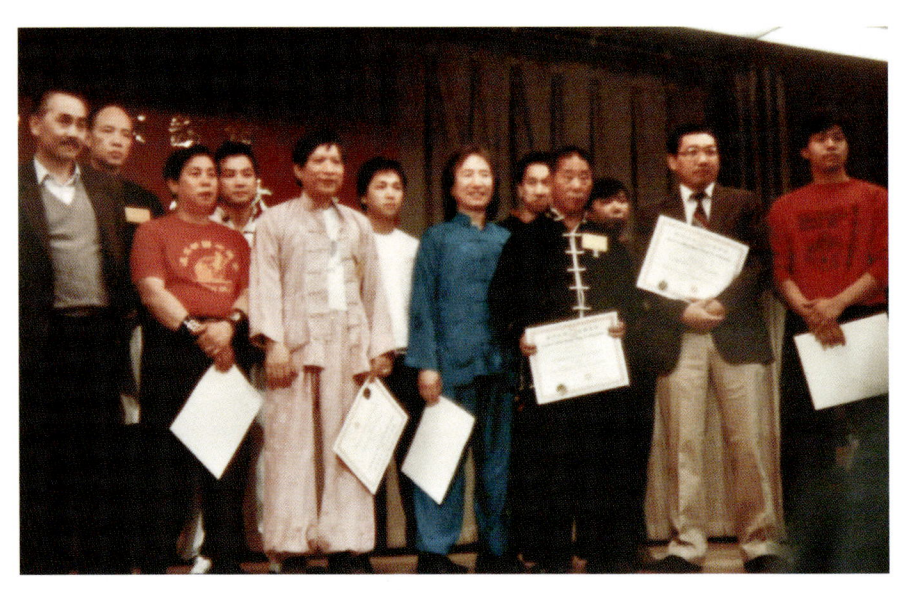

All Kung-fu Masters Exhibition 1988. *Front Row (from left):* 1. Ng Wai Hong (Fu Jow Pai); 2. Wan Chi Ming (Hung Gar); 3. Kenny Gong (Hsing–I); 4. C K Chu; 5. Chan Tai San (Lama Pai); 6. Fong Ji Yu (Fu Jow Pai). *Back Row:* Tak Eng (Fu Jow Pai) between C K Chu and Chan Tai San.

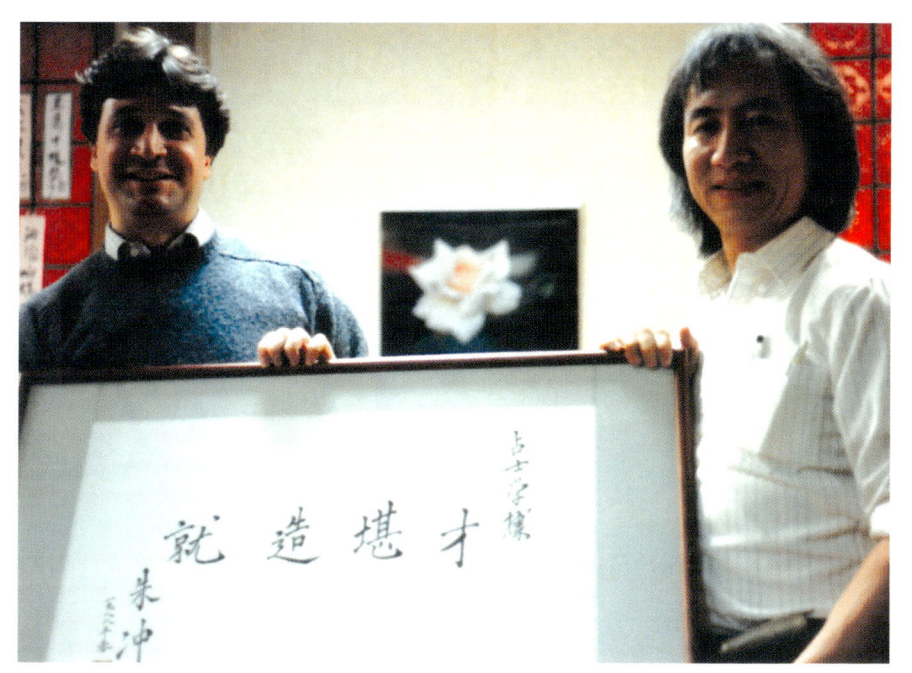

Master Chu presents a commemorative calligraphy to Jim Borrelli for his assistance on *The Book of Nei Kung*.

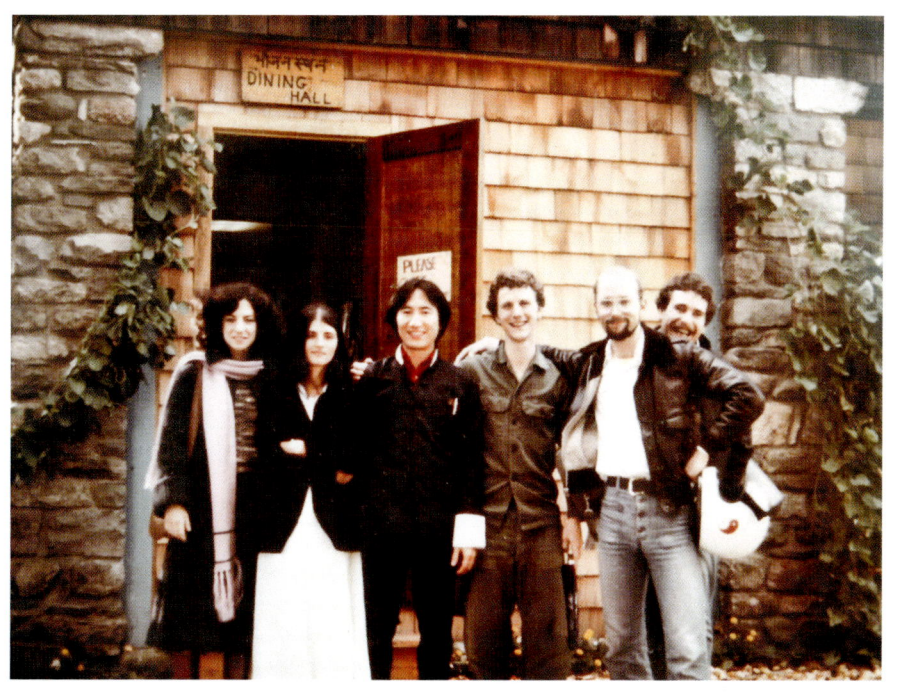

For many years, Master Chu took students on retreat to Ananda Ashram in Monroe, NY. In the group picture, note that John Sharamko (first on right in front) helped with *The Book of Nei Kung*.

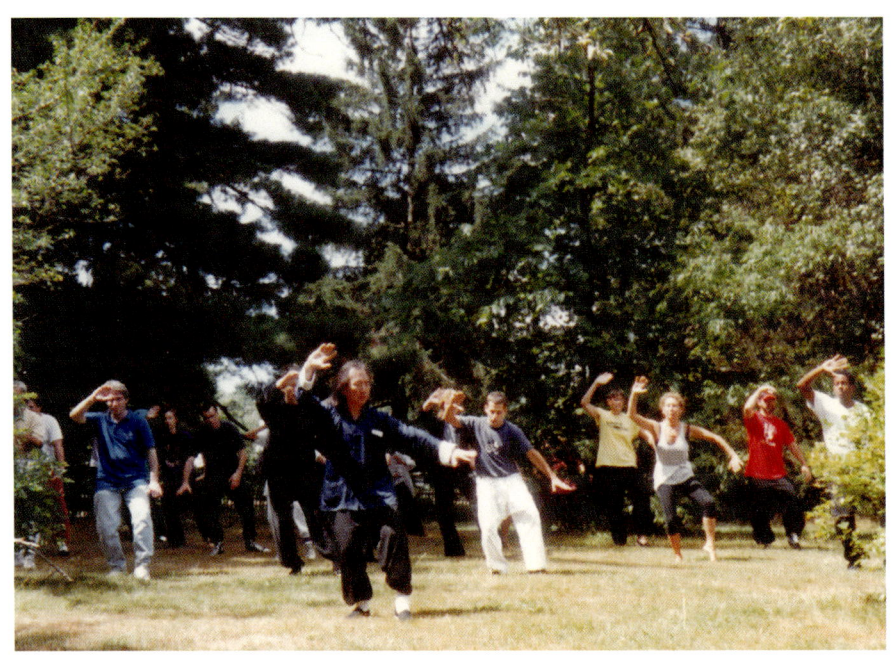

Students doing the form as a group during the Monroe Retreat.

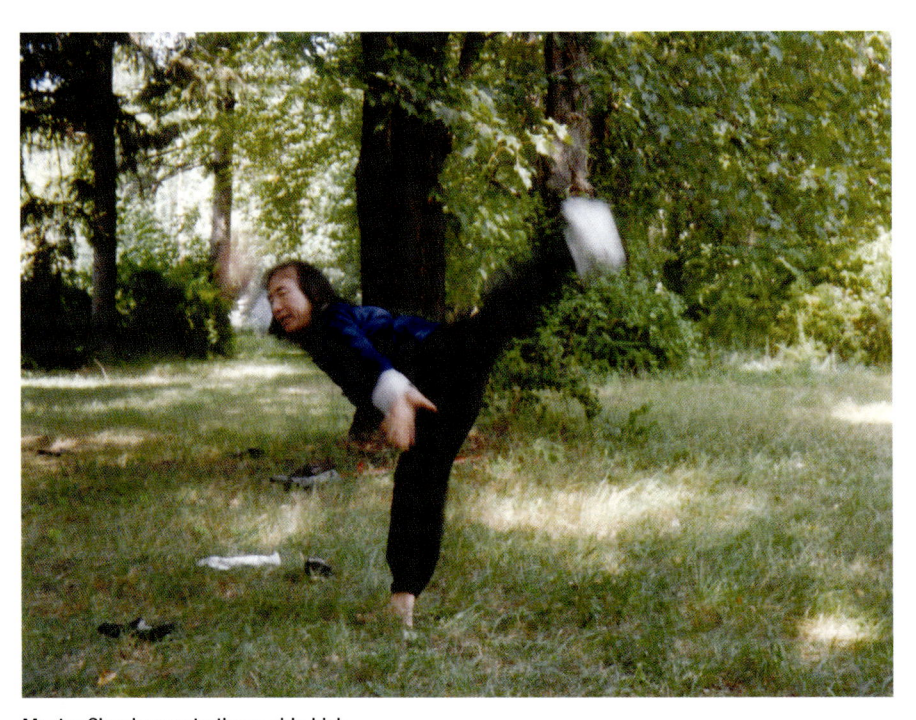

Master Chu demonstrating a side kick.

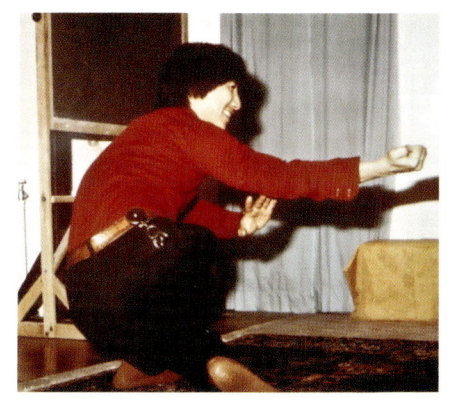

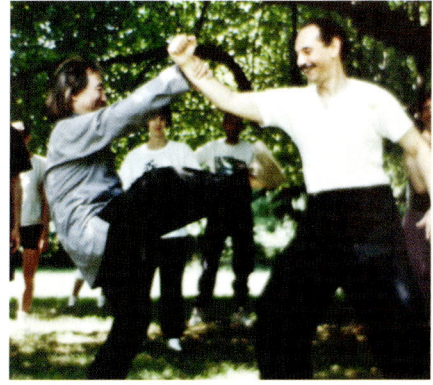

Master Chu demonstrating a Buddhist Fist posture and a heel kick at the Monroe Retreat.

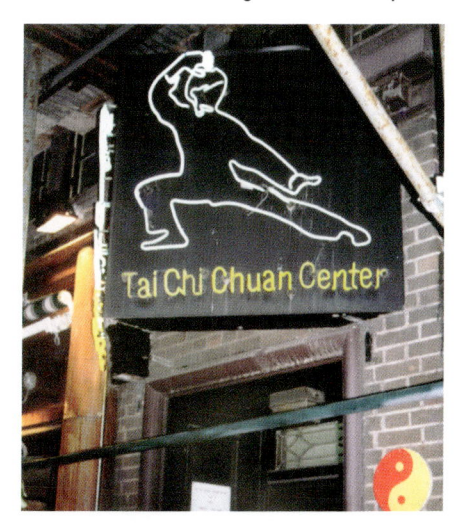

In 1989, the school moved to 125 West 43rd Street.

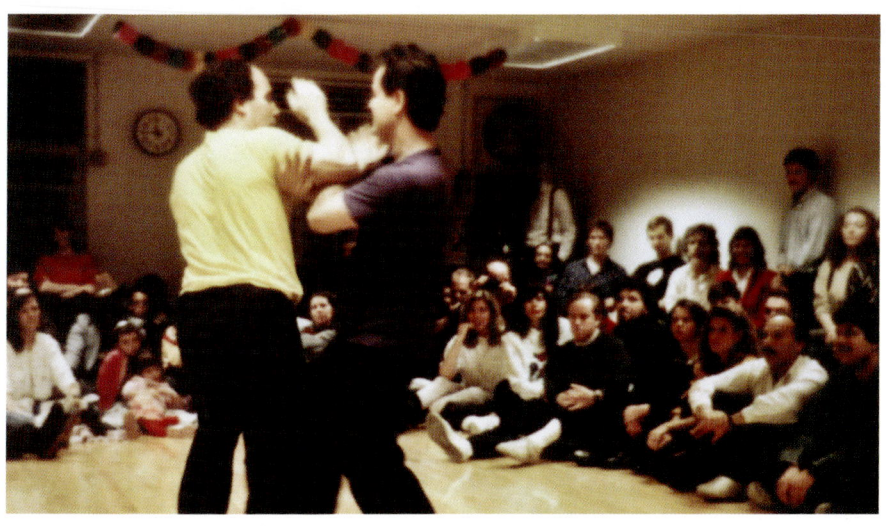

To celebrate the school's new location, we had a housewarming party with demonstrations and a banquet in March 1990.

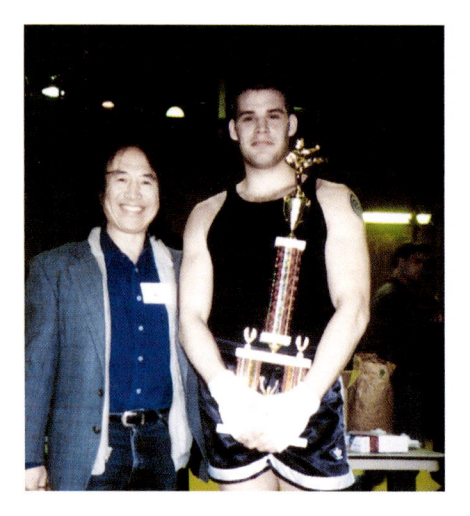

In 1995, Hugh Marlowe won two champion titles in two separate tournaments during the same weekend.

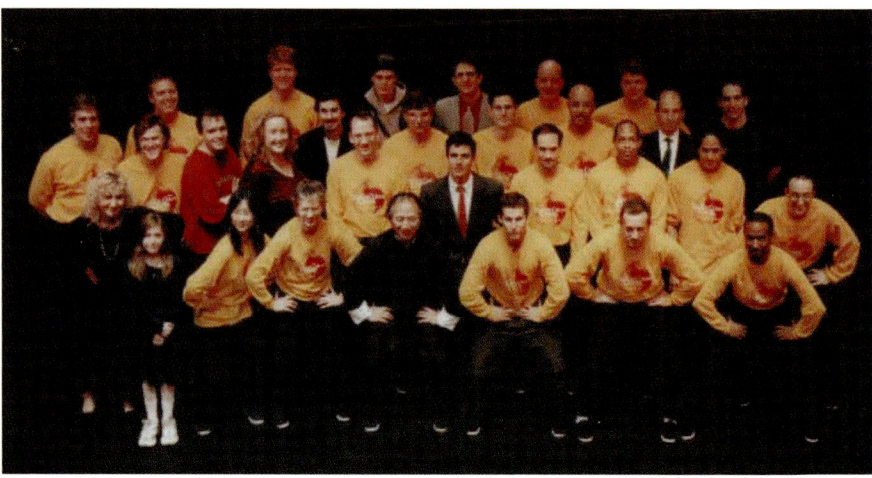

To kick off the new non-profit, Tai Chi Chuan Center, we put together a benefit performance at Pace University, November 11, 2000.

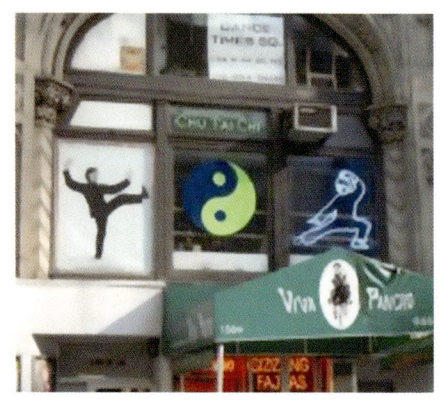

In 2001, we moved to our current location at 156 West 44th Street.

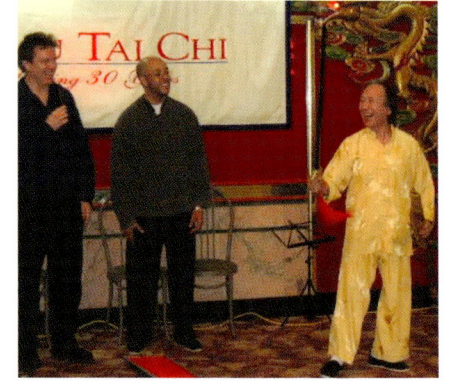

In honor of Chu Tai Chi's 30th Anniversary, students present Master Chu with an honorary sword.

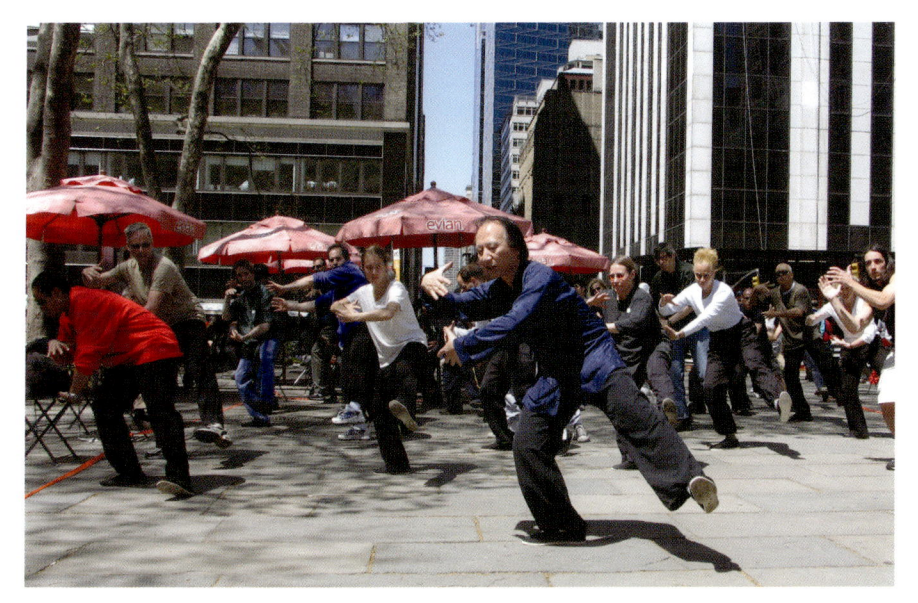

The Tai Chi Chuan Center's purpose is to educate the broader public about tai chi. The board members and supporters believe that, like access to healthy air, food and water, it is essential that people have access to healthy exercise. Thus, the Tai Chi Chuan Center Board has made possible free Eternal Spring Classes in Bryant Park, which served nearly 2000 student hours in 2010 alone. Architect and former board member, Gary Jacquemin, was instrumental in designing the interiors of the last two schools. Current board members include Nathaniel Wice, Lee Velta, Dan Zegibe, Norman Ellis, Anita Durst, and Dan Nash.

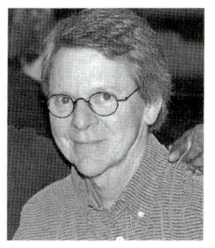

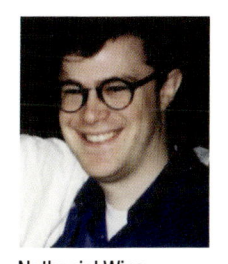

Gary Jacquemin

Nathaniel Wice

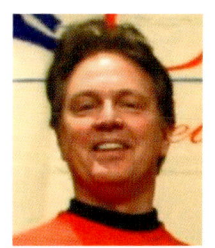

Lee Velta

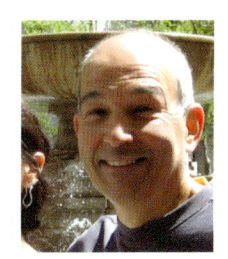

Dan Zegibe

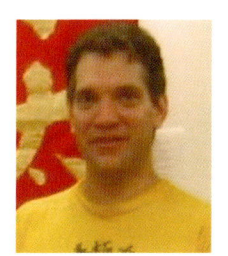

Dan Nash

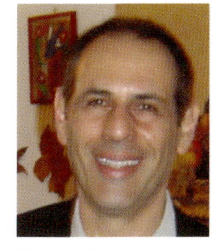

Norman Ellis

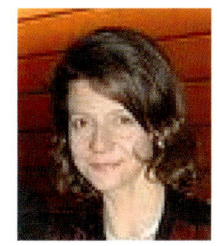

Anita Durst

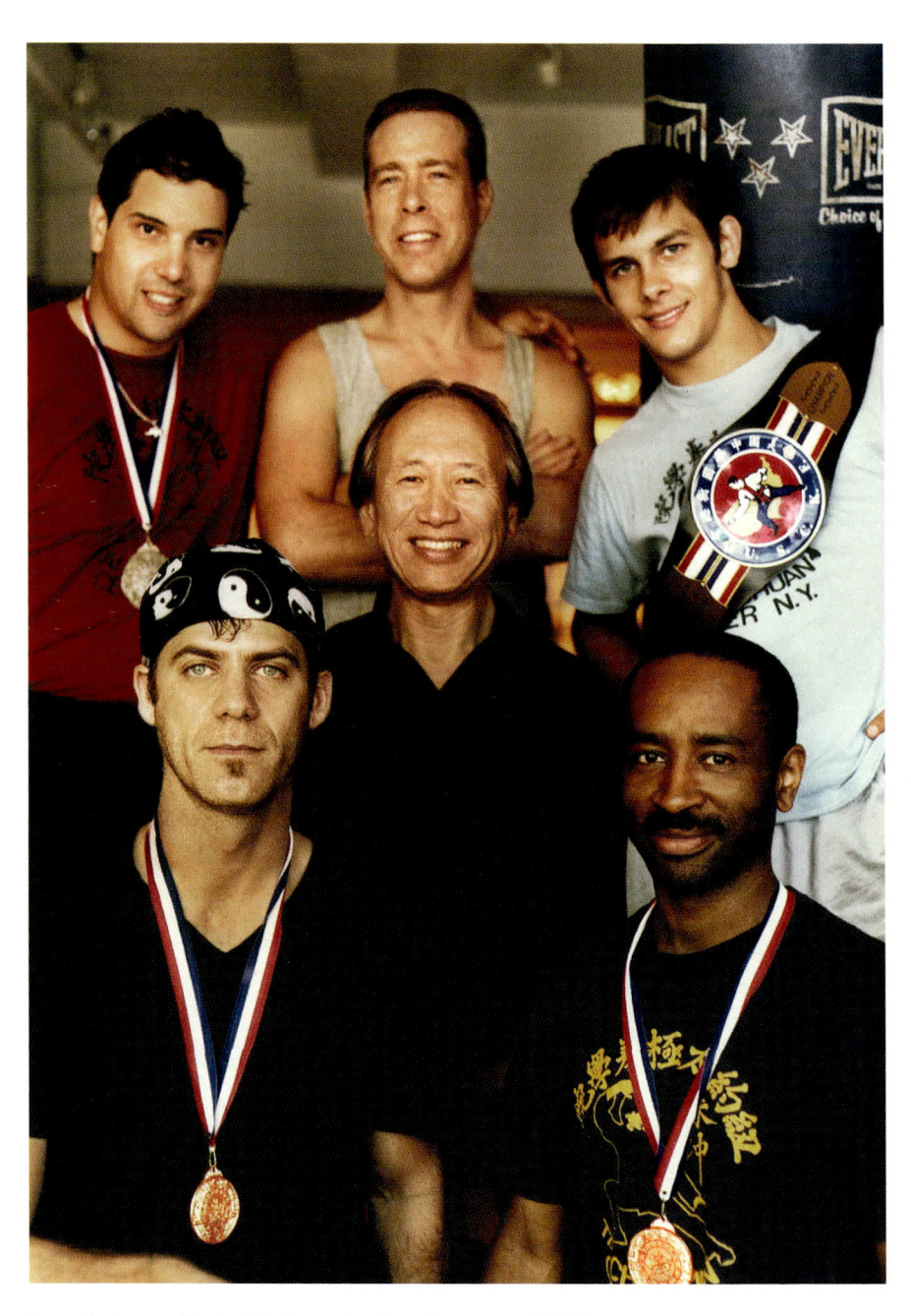

For several years, Master Chu (center) took students to the USKF Tournament in Baltimore: Master Chu surrounded by student champions and assistants of 2005: (clockwise from lower left) Jesse Shadoan, Rene Gonzalez, Lindsey Horner, John Signoriello, Hyland Harris.

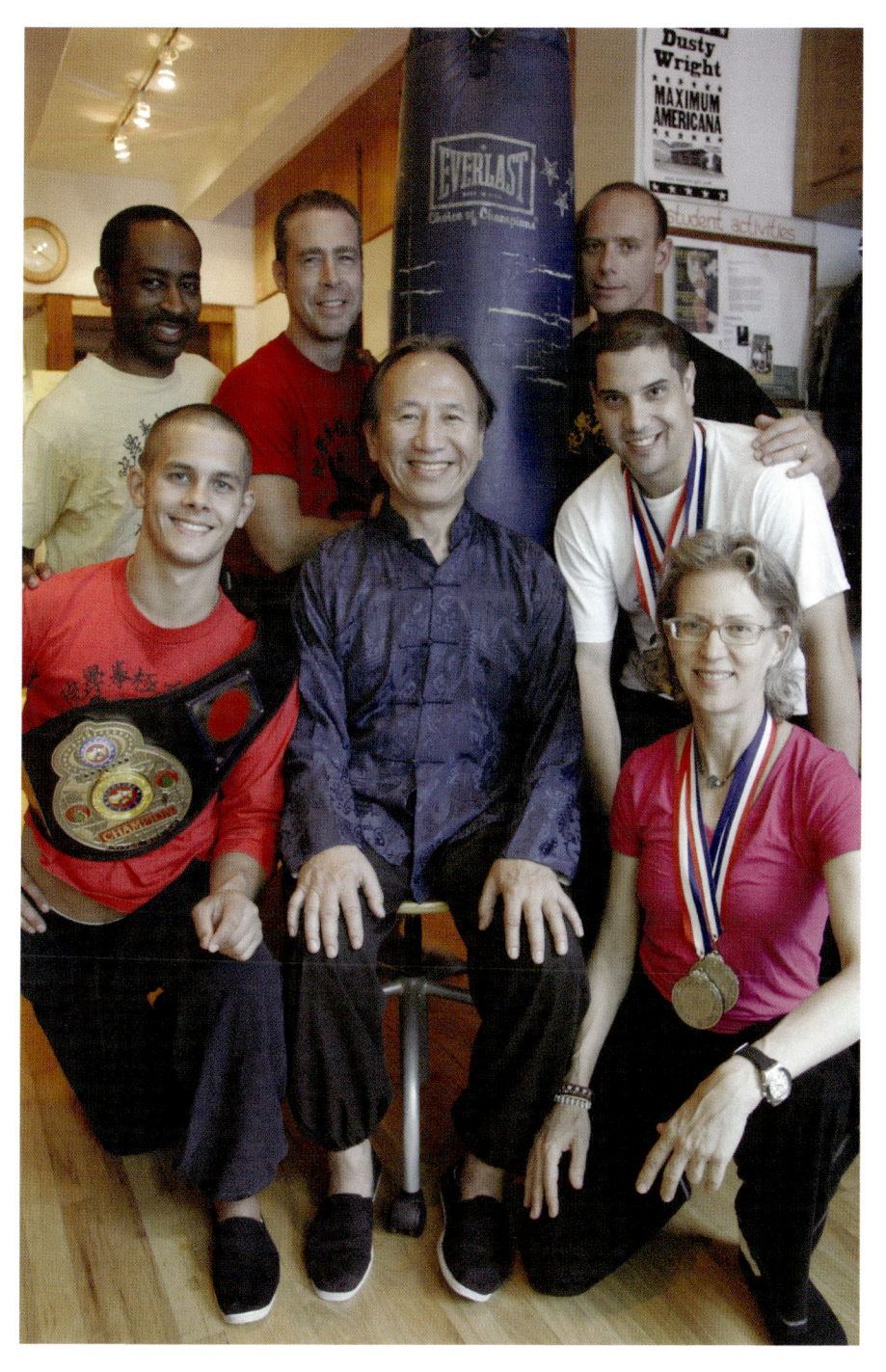

Master Chu (center) and student fighters of 2006 with assistants: (clockwise from lower left) John Signoriello, Hyland Harris, Lindsey Horner, Jeff Pastoressa, Rene Gonzalez, and Kate Wasilewski.

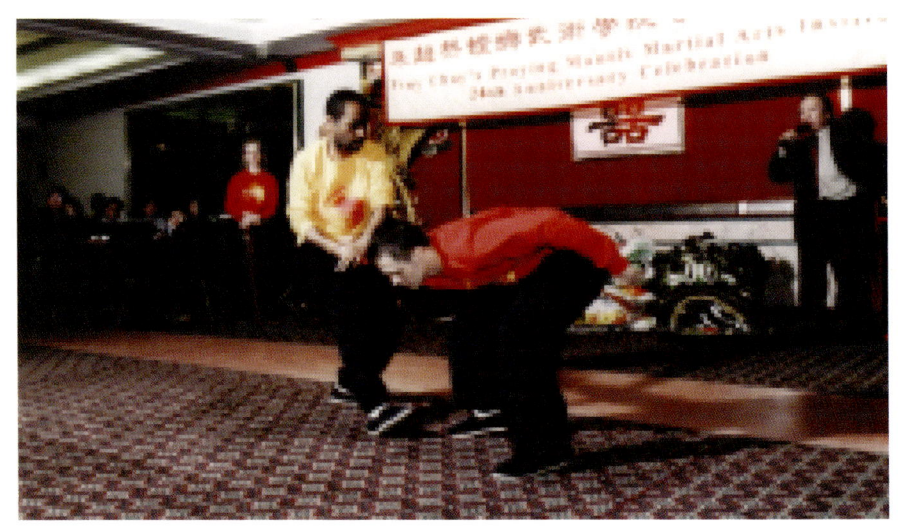

Hyland Harris (yellow shirt) proved the system even works for someone in their late 30s. Despite committing himself to the tournament only a month beforehand, he did not need to alter the training he was already doing. He went to Baltimore and faced someone who was almost half his age, a bigger and stronger hard-style shaolin stylist. Hyland took him down several times, uprooted him and won by knockout.

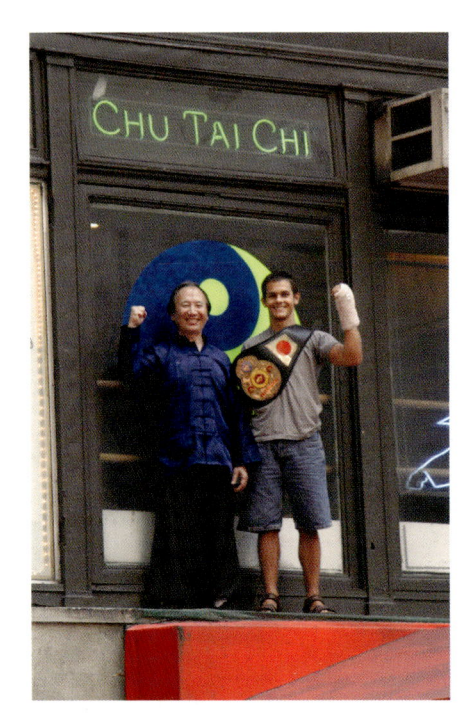

Master Chu and John Signoriello (with the competitor of the year belt over his shoulder) pose on the outside of the school window over 44th Street.

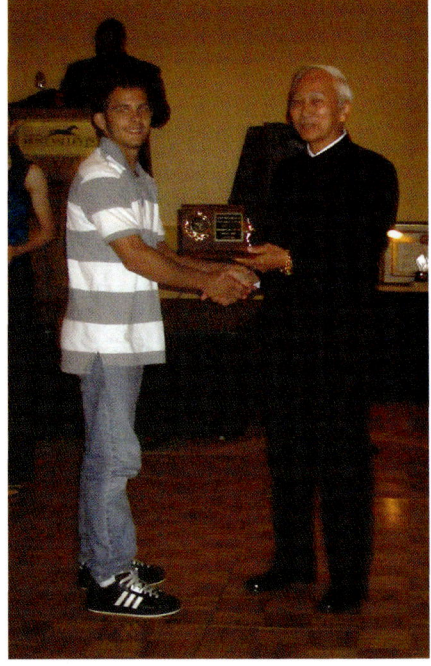

Master Huang, president of the USCKF, presents John Signoriello with the 'competitor of the year' award, their highest honor.

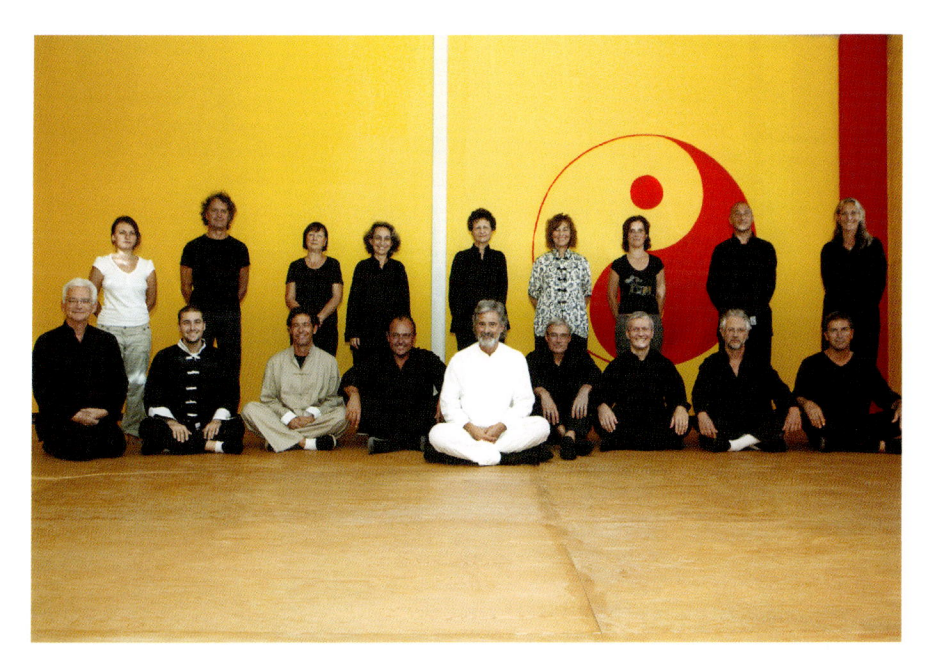

Master Chu's tai chi has spread throughout the world. Master Riccardo Consani (center, in white uniform) teaches in Italy at Tai Chi Chuan Centro di Studio Lucca.

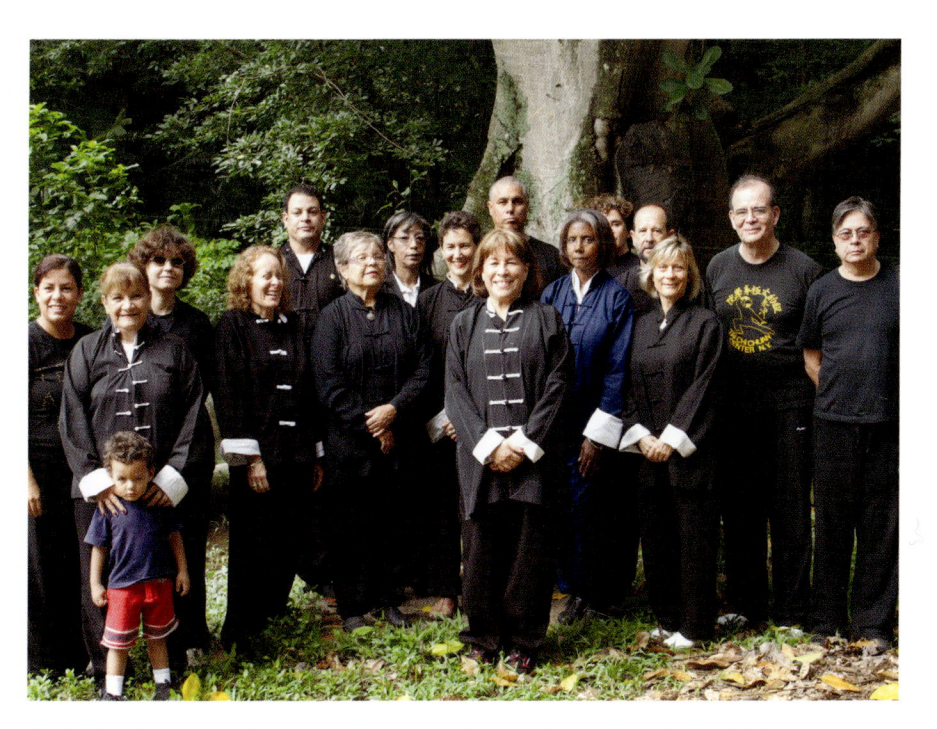

Master Eka Marquez (front row, center) teaches in Caracas, Venezuela, at the Tai Chi Chuan Centro de Estudio.

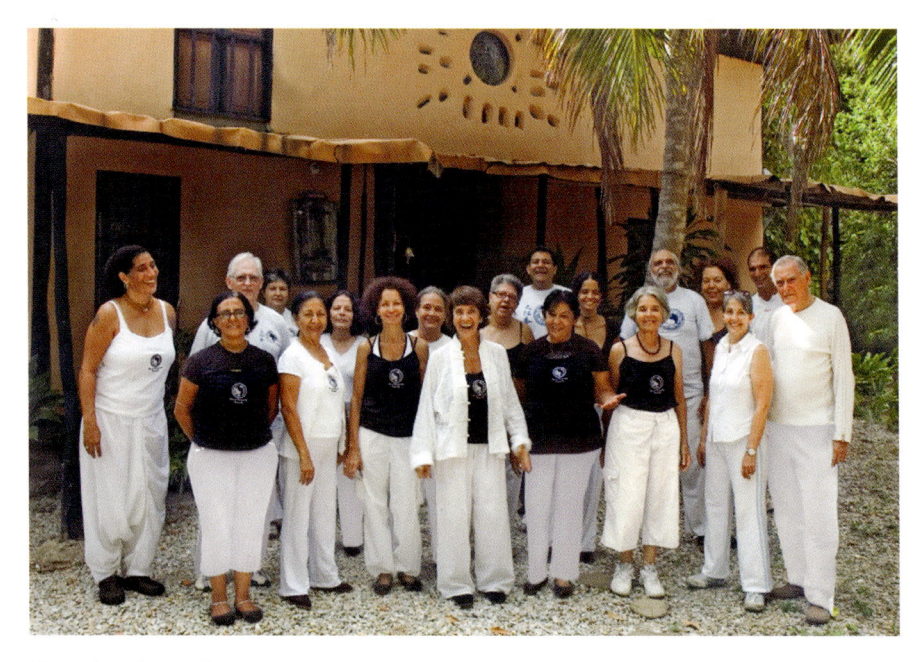

Master Ines Gomez (front row, wearing white jacket) teaches tai chi at the Tai Chi Chuan Center on Margarita Island.

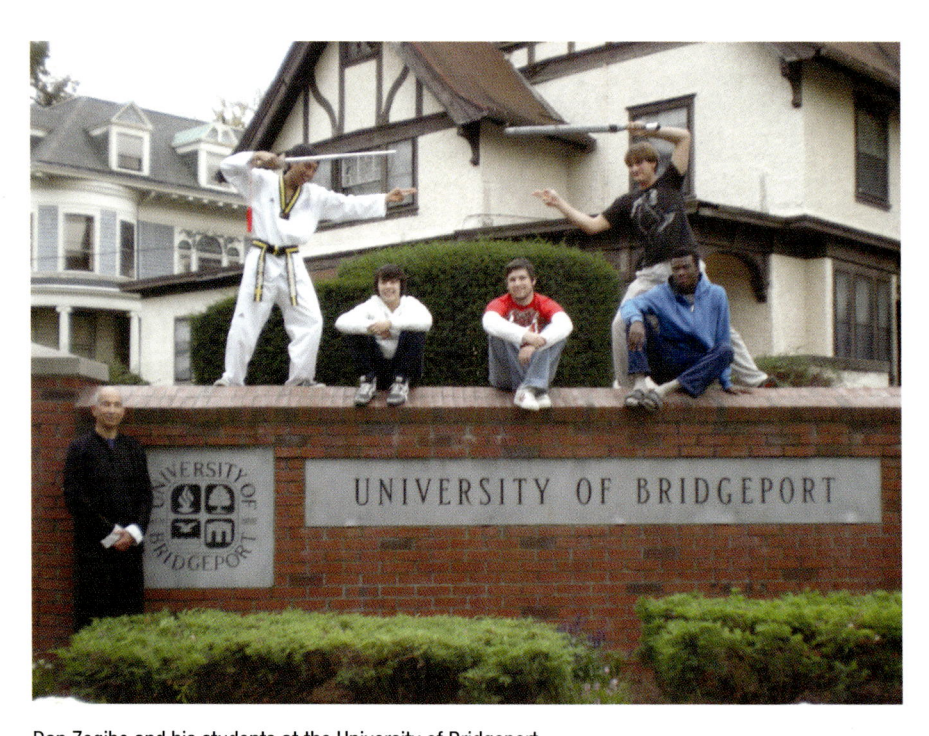

Dan Zegibe and his students at the University of Bridgeport.

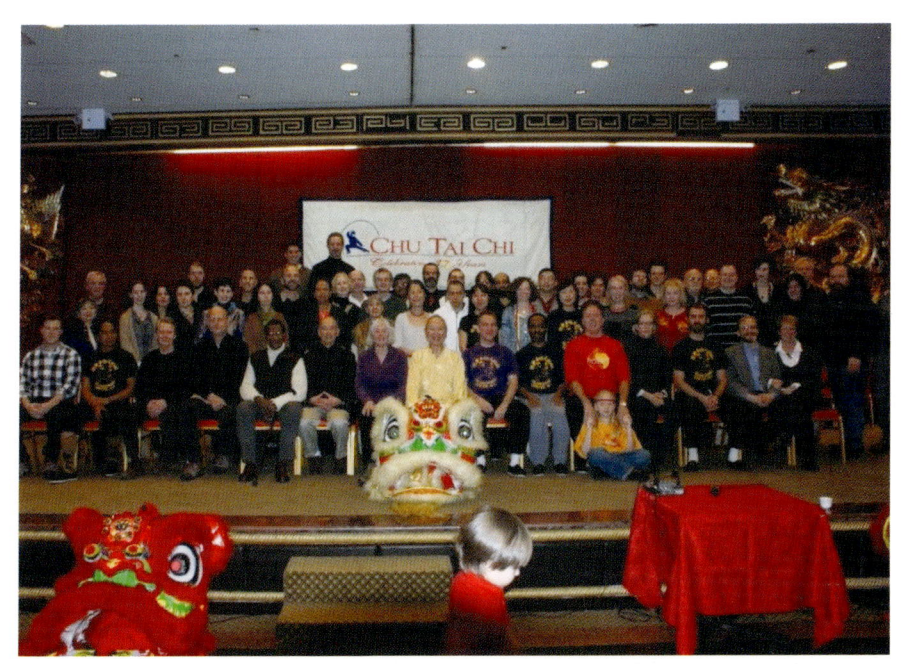

Master Chu and the students of CK Chu Tai Chi at the 2010 Chinese New Year Banquet.

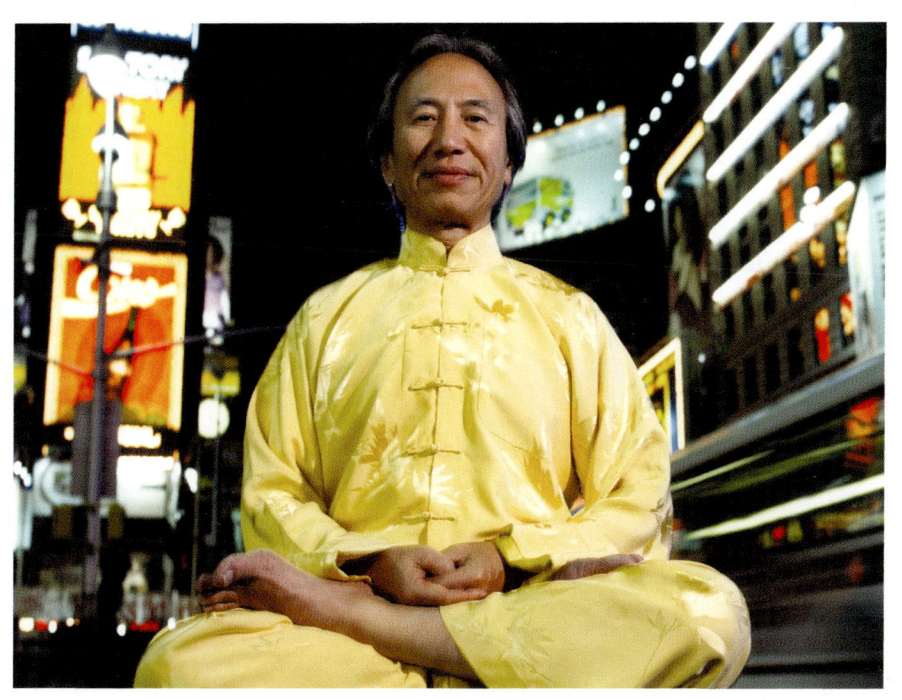

CK Chu Tai Chi is an oasis of calm in the midst of the glittering lights and crowd of Times Square, crossroads of the world.

CK Chu Tai Chi teaching assistants and Eternal Spring teachers: Hyland Harris, John Signorelli, Ben Ho, Dan Zegibe, Dan Nash, Jim Hicks, Steve Miller, Alex Kamlet, John Van Wettering, Kate Wasilewski, Evan Wilson; Jeremy W. Hubbell, Sivan Shar, John Lake, Jesse Shadoan, Dora Chu, Rob Hoffman, Gabor Reisinger, Akiko Hikota, Kathleen Keck, Pietro Sabatino, Martin Andrews, Dick Esterle, Carlton Holmes, Mike Davey, Justin Tentler and Joseph Barbarino.

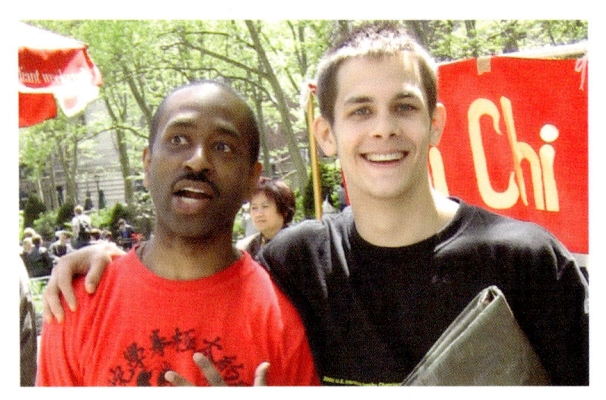

Hyland Harris & John Signorelli

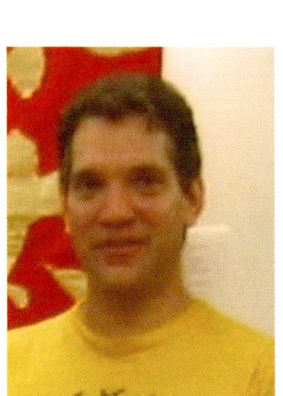

Ben Ho

Dan Zegibe

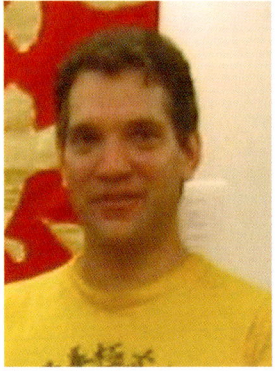

Dan Nash

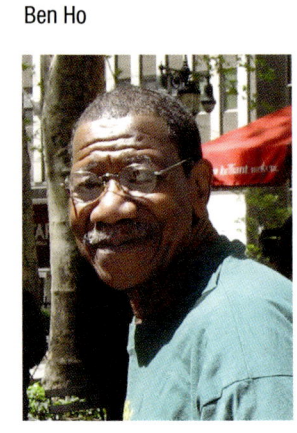

Jim Hicks

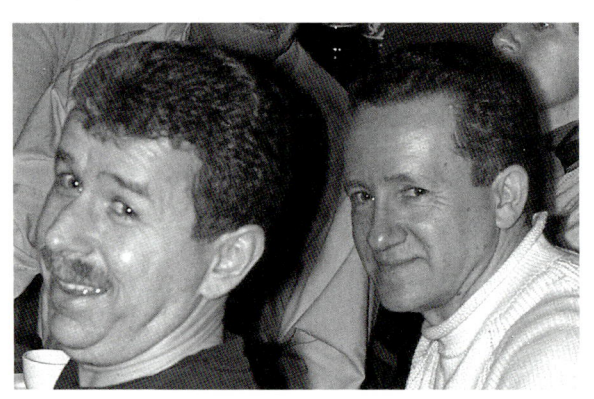

Steve Miller and Alex Kamlet

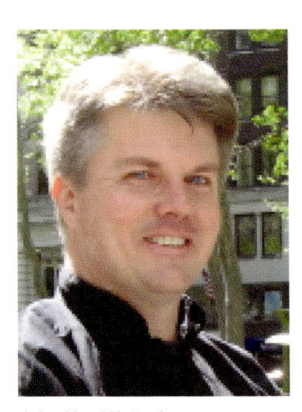

John Van Wettering

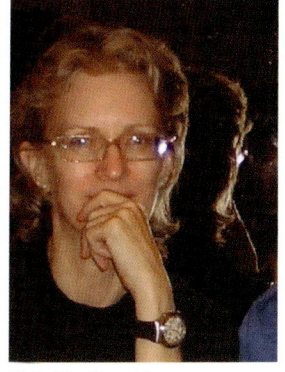

Kate Wasilewski

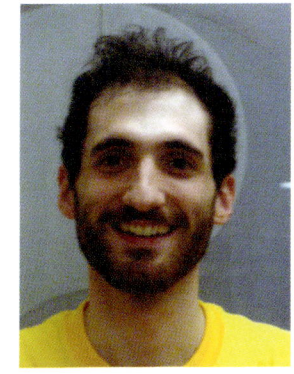

Evan Wilson

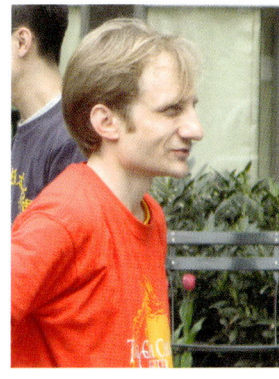

Jeremy W. Hubbell

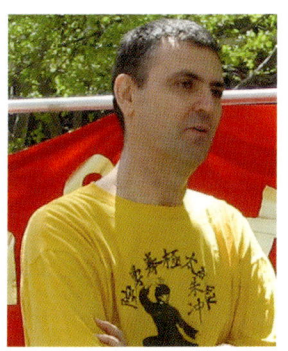

Sivan Shar

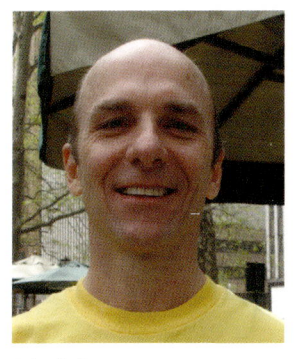

John Lake

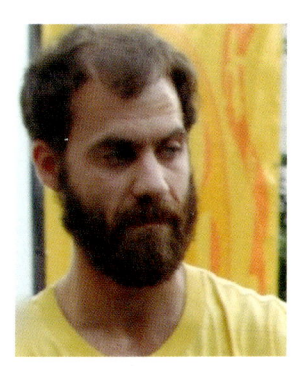

Jesse Shadoan

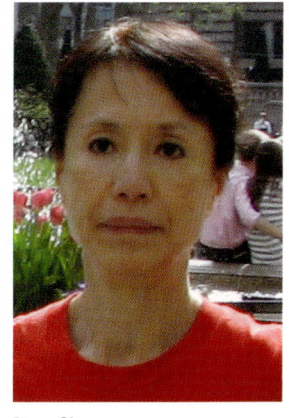

Dora Chu

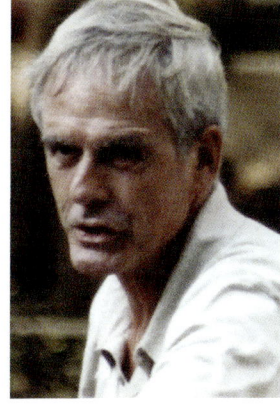

Rob Hoffman

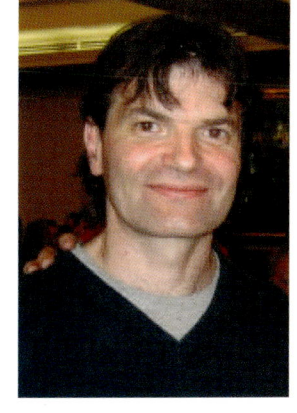

Gabor Reisinger

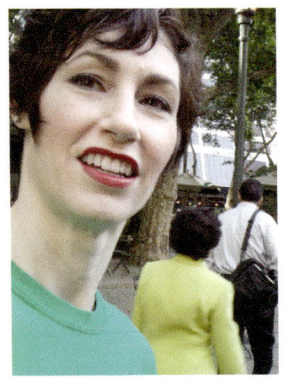

Kathleen Keck

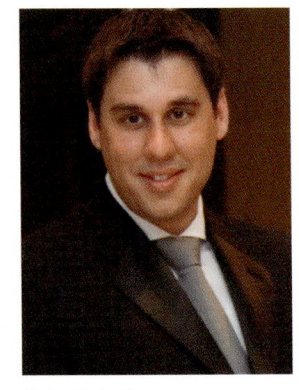

Pietro Sabatino

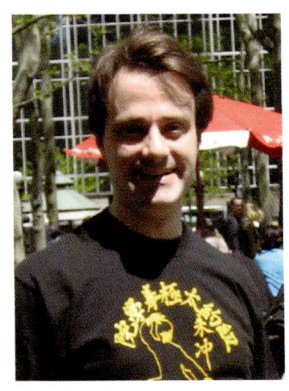

Martin Andrews

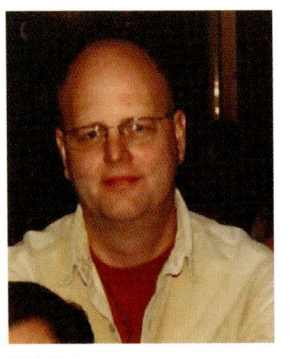

Dick Esterle

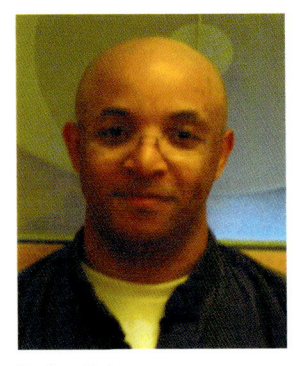

Carlton Holmes

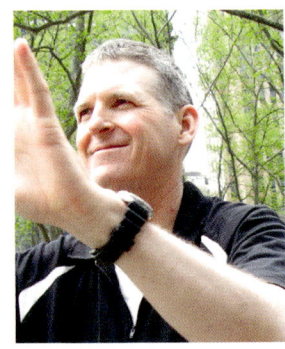

Mike Davey

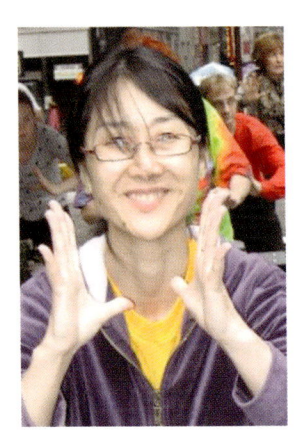

Akiko Hikota

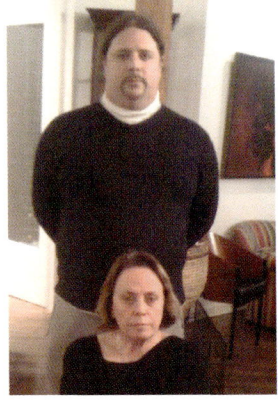

Justin Tentler, Eternal Spring instructor, with his mother, Dr. Adrienne Harris. Dr. Adrienne Harris is a long-time generous supporter of the Tai Chi Chuan Center's outreach program.

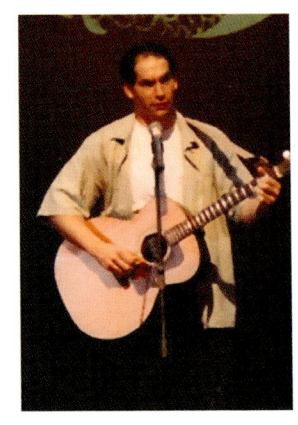

Joseph Barbarino

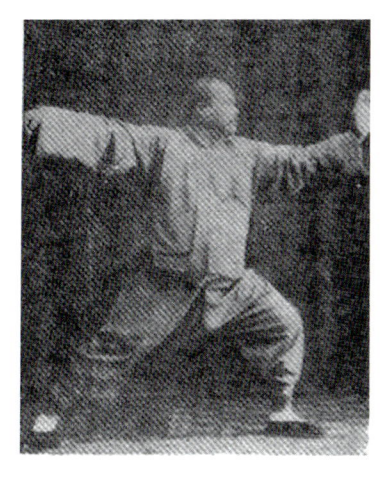

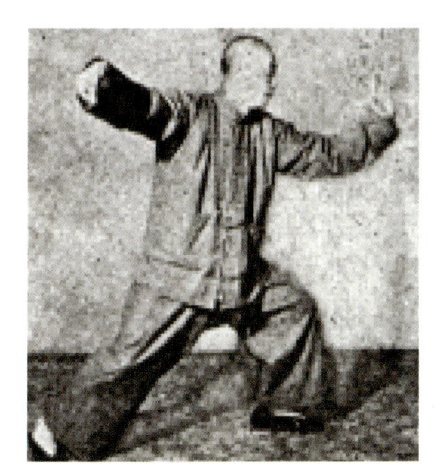

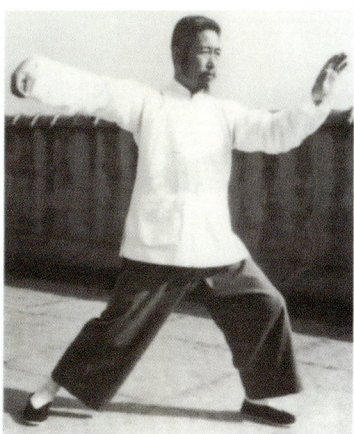

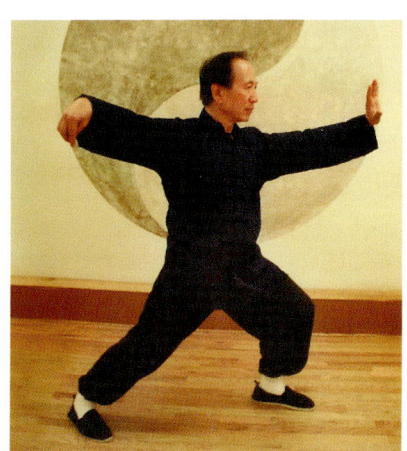

Single Whip is unique to tai chi. Here, Single Whip is demonstrated by Yang Cheng-fu, Tung Ying-chieh, Chen Man-ch'ing, and CK Chu.

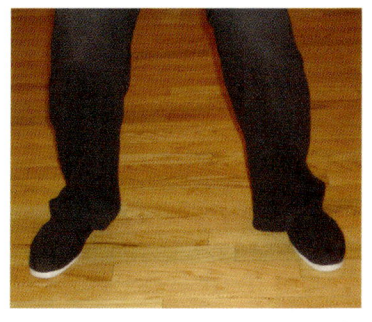

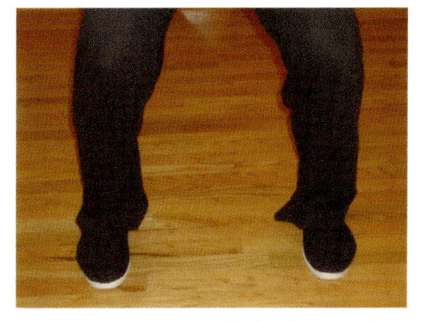

In tai chi, whether doing the form, *chi kung* or *nei kung*, there is a correct body alignment. In Horse Stance, the knees should be over the toes. The first image (left) shows incorrect knee alignment, the second picture (right) shows the correct alignment (see questions 2.8 & 4.8).

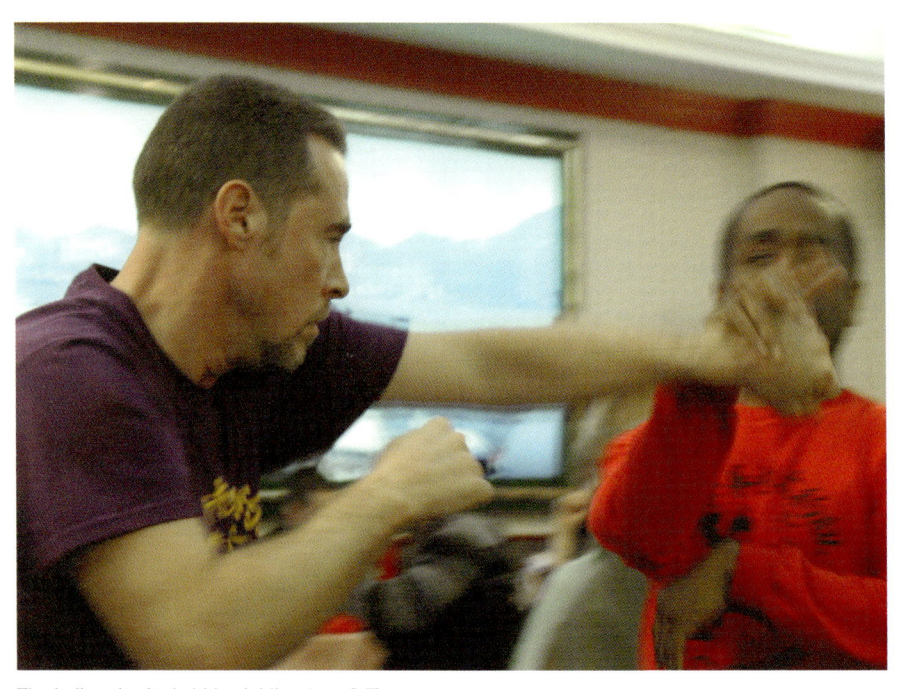

The hallmark of tai chi is yielding (see 3.7).
Students demonstrate yielding drills at the New Year Banquet.

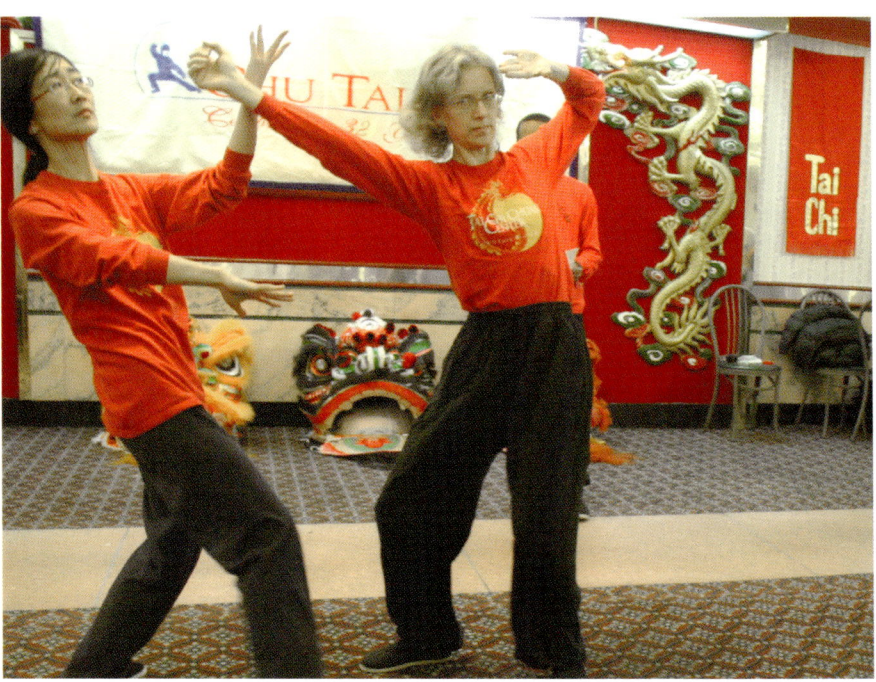

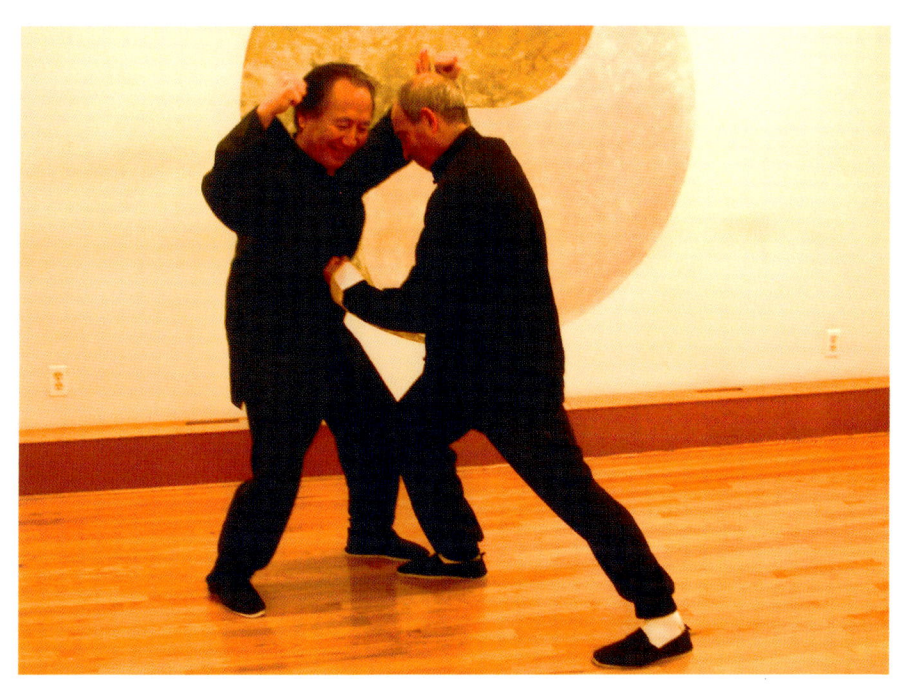

Master Chu demonstrates the power of "iron-vest" (or nei kung) training by taking a punch to the stomach (see 6.2).

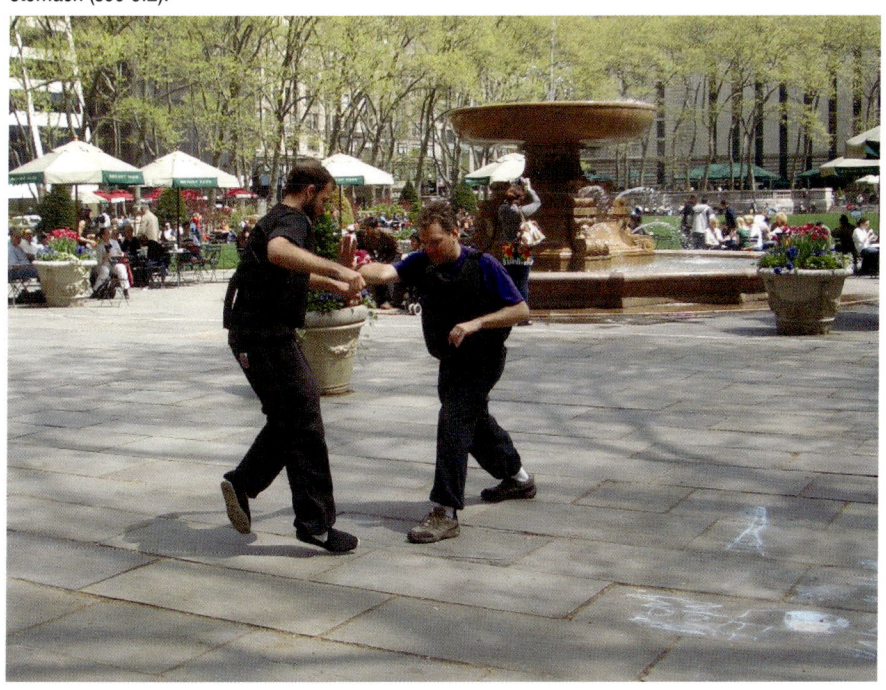

Students demonstrate the power of tai chi for World Tai Chi Day.

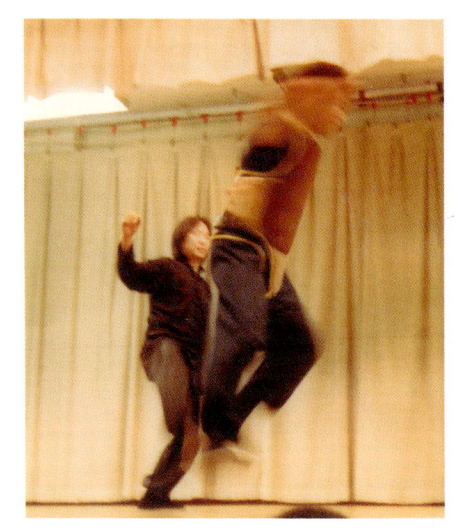

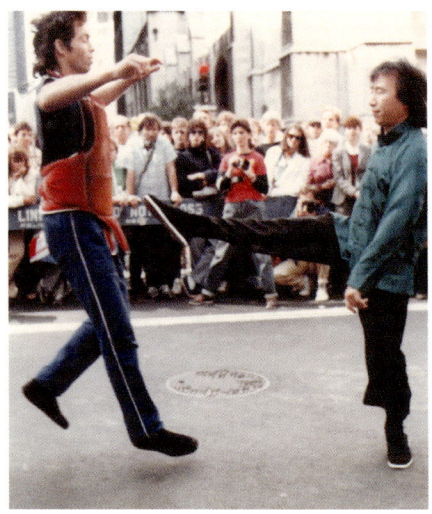

Master Chu demonstrates the striking power of tai chi. In these two he demonstrates kicks.

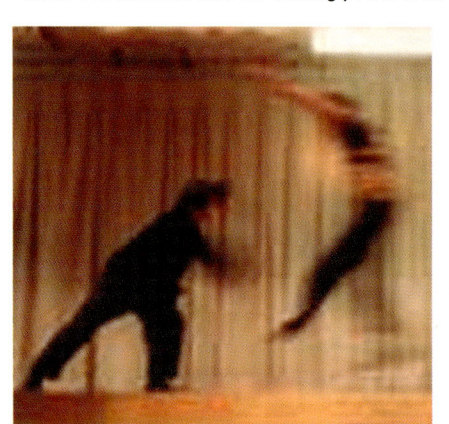

A demonstration of Brush Knee.

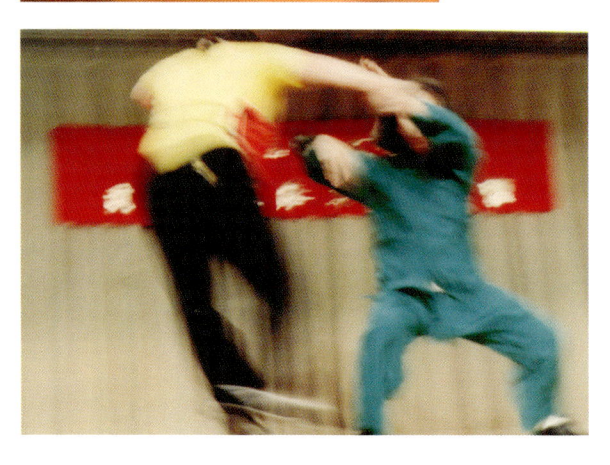

Master Chu demonstration of Grasp Bird's Tail.

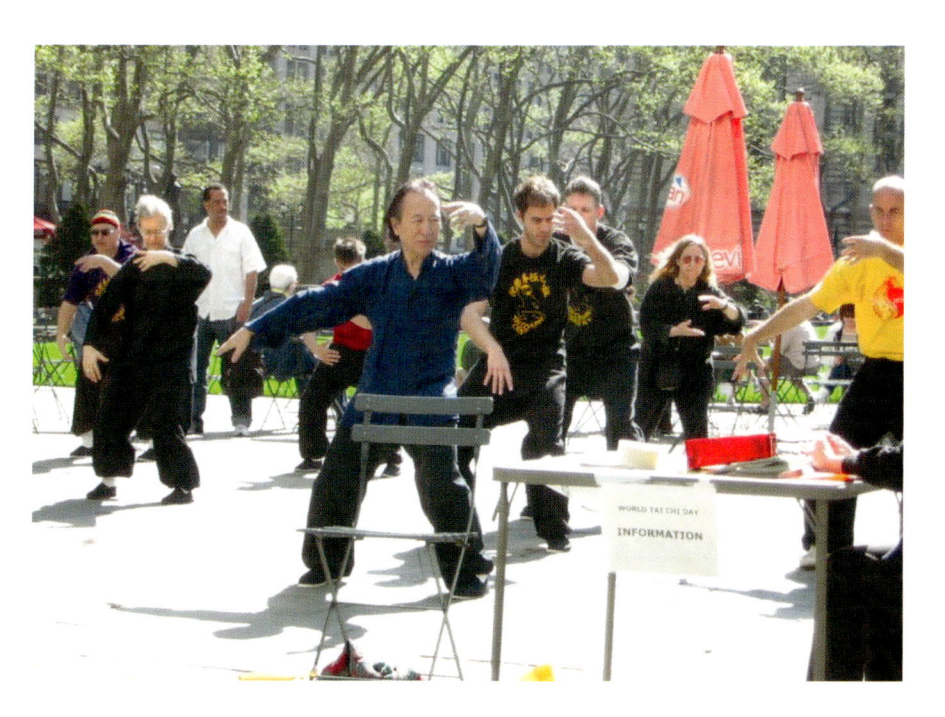

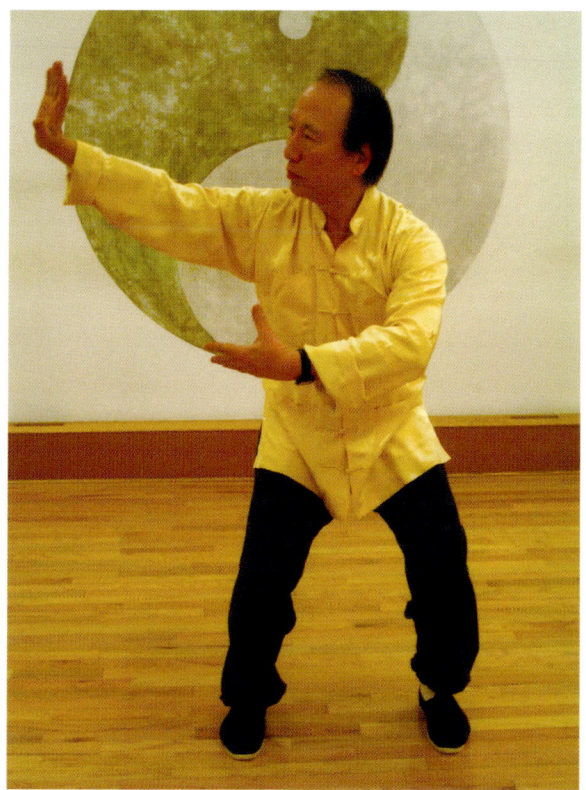

Master Chu and students demonstrate Wave Hands, which is a Silk-Reeling exercise (see 3.27).

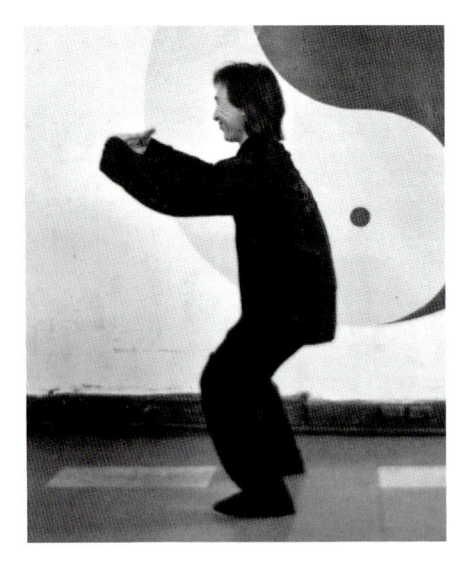

Master Chu demonstrates the Horse Stance (see chapter 6). As noted in 4.8 and 4.9, his back is round and his chest is concave.

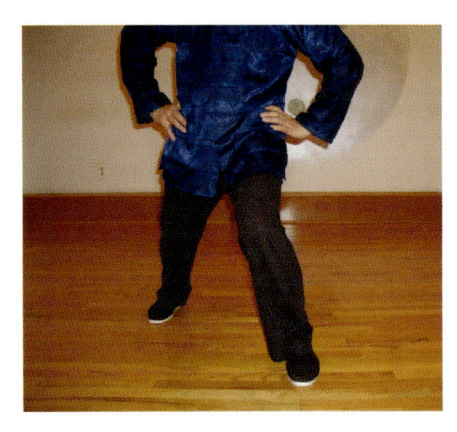

Maintaining alignment throughout the form is vital (4.9-4.12).

The picture at left shows incorrect alignment.

The pictures below show correct alignment for the Bow and Arrow Stance.

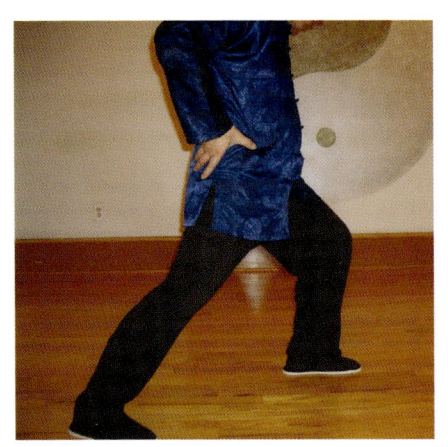

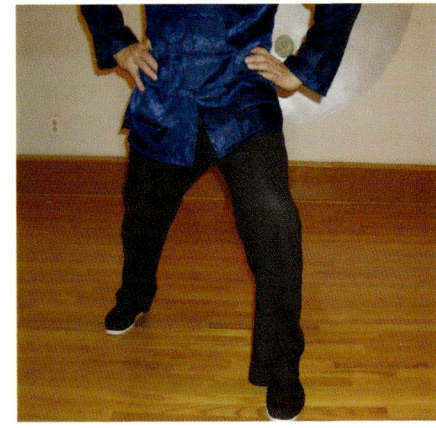

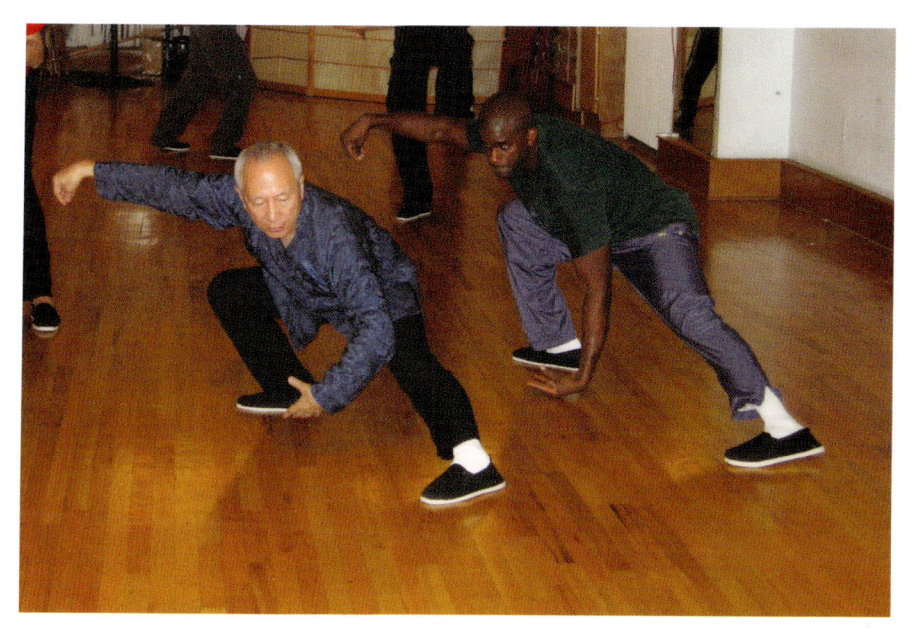

At CK Chu Tai Chi, the form is taught in the traditional way, one-on-one, by Master Chu or one of his students. Each movement must be internalized by the student at his or her own pace. Above, Master Chu is teaching Snake Creeps Down. Below, Master Chu's student, Dan Nash, is teaching the opening of the form during a Tai Chi Class at the school.

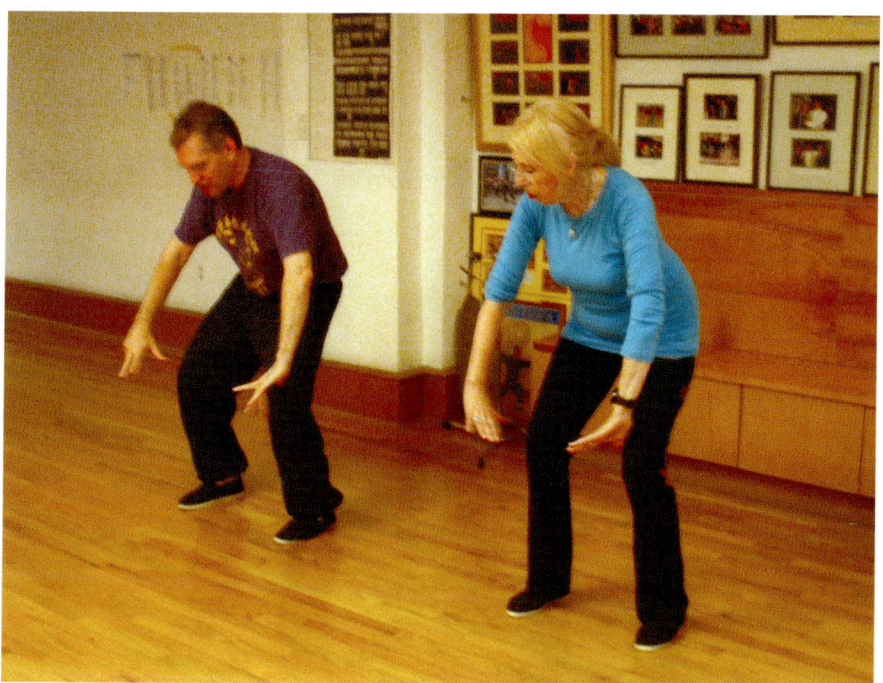

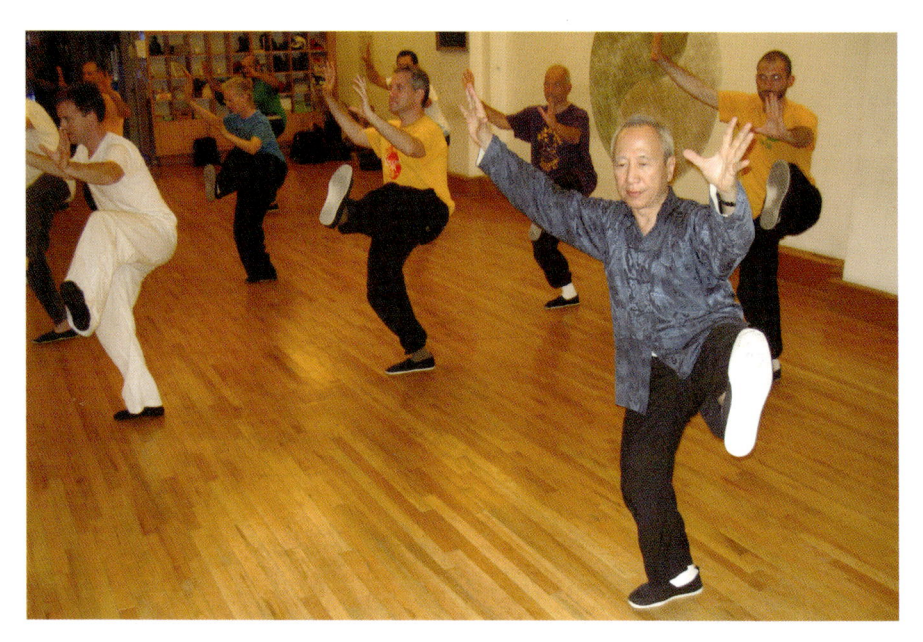

Tai Chi is a fighting art and at CK Chu Tai Chi, students who have learned the form can take Fighting Classes where they learn how to apply the moves. In these two photos, Master Chu leads the students of a Fighting Class in the form.

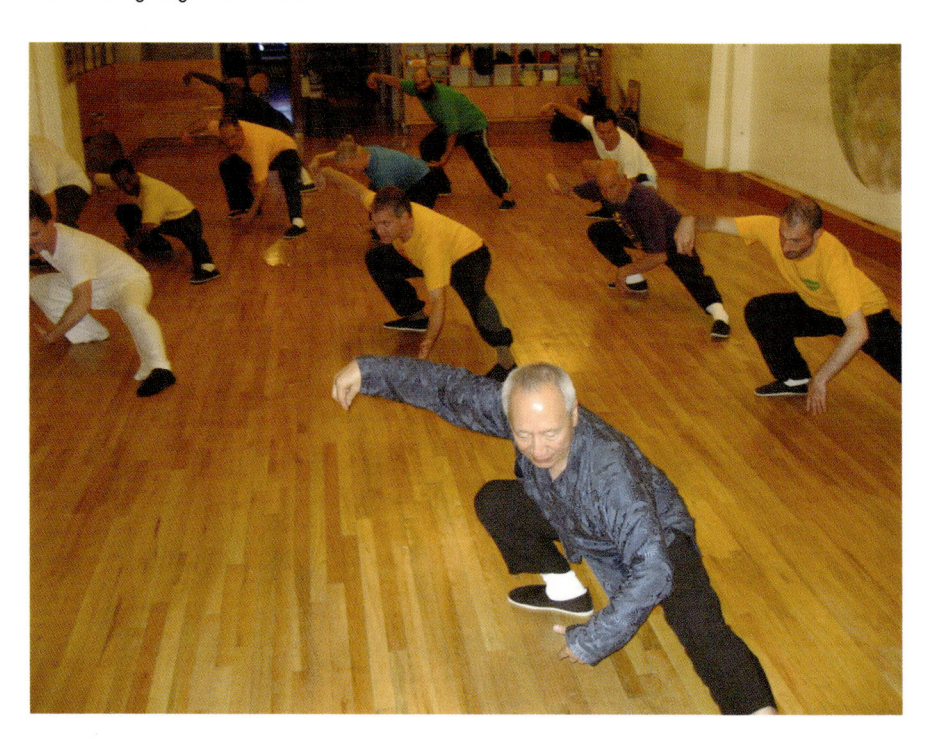

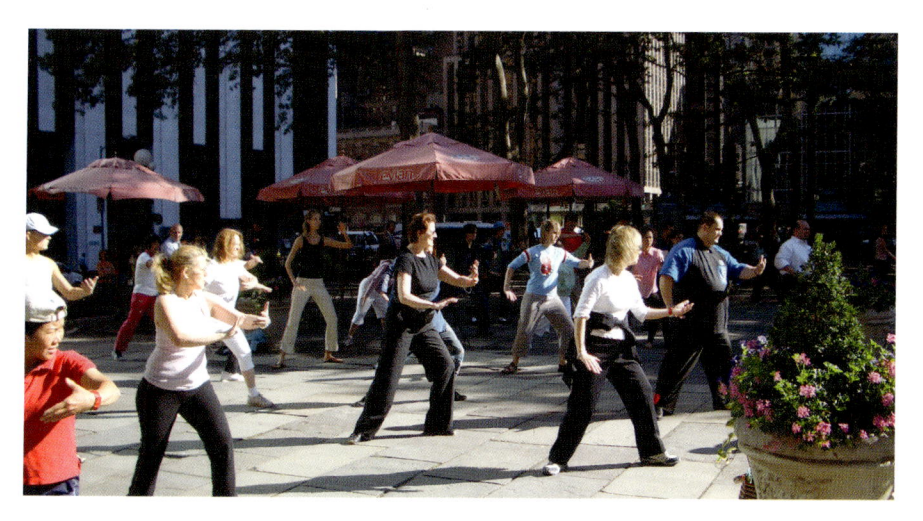

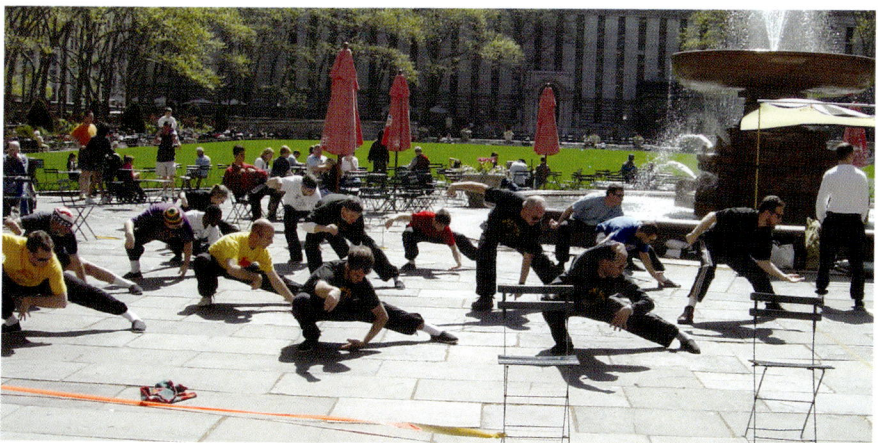

Students doing the tai chi form in Bryant Park.

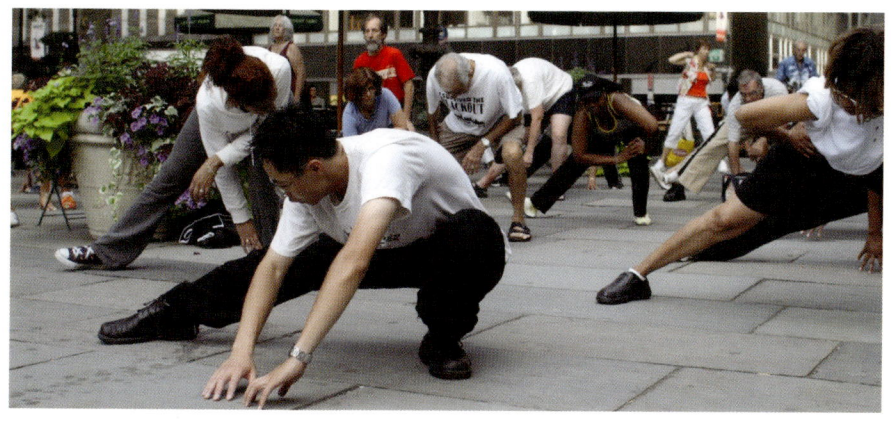

Shifting Frog, an Eternal Spring exercise, opens the qua (discussed in 5.18).

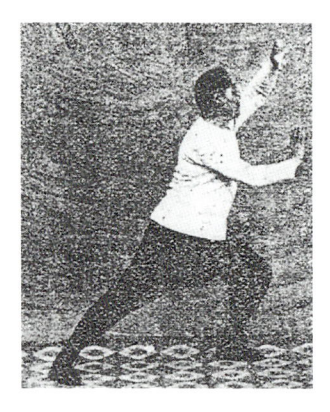

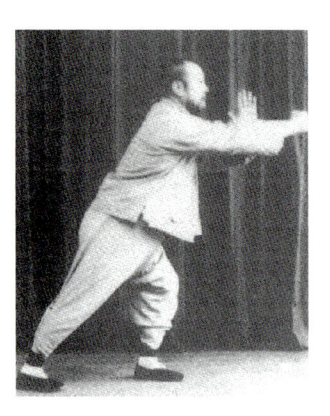

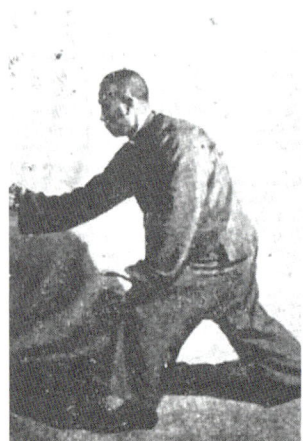

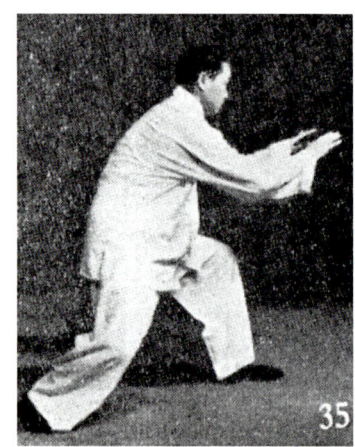

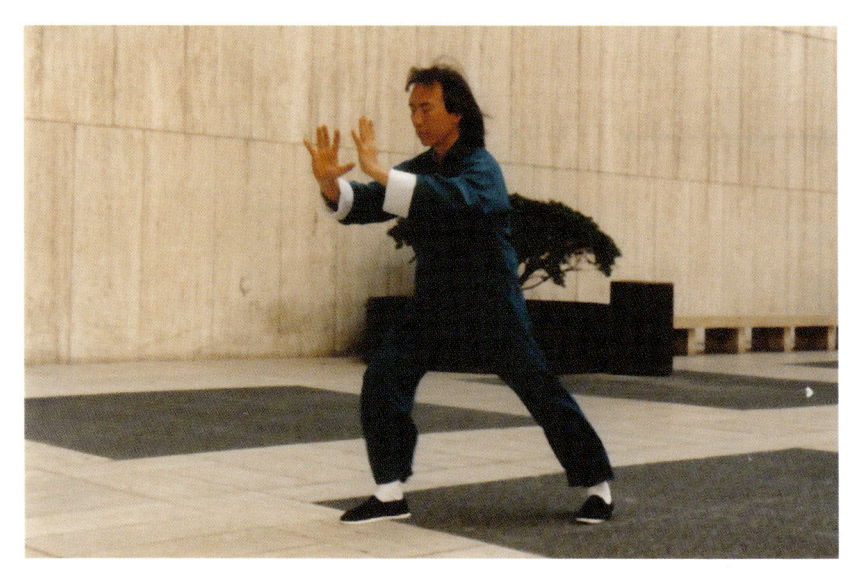

Question 5.3 refers to a common misconception about the meaning of 'leaning forward'. In this series, you can see masters doing the form with a straight back and leaning forward: (from left to right : Yang Cheng-fu , Wu Jianquan, Tung Ying-chieh, Dong Hu Ling, and CK Chu.)

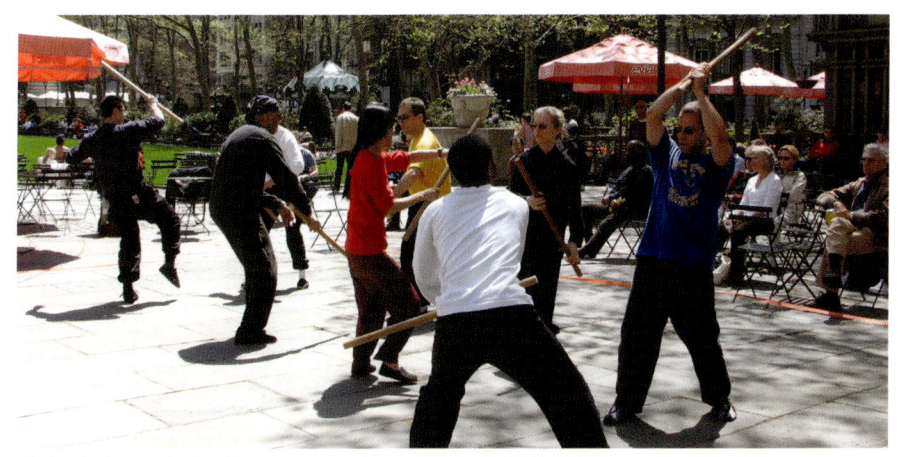

Students demonstrating Two-person Stick Form on World Tai Chi Day.

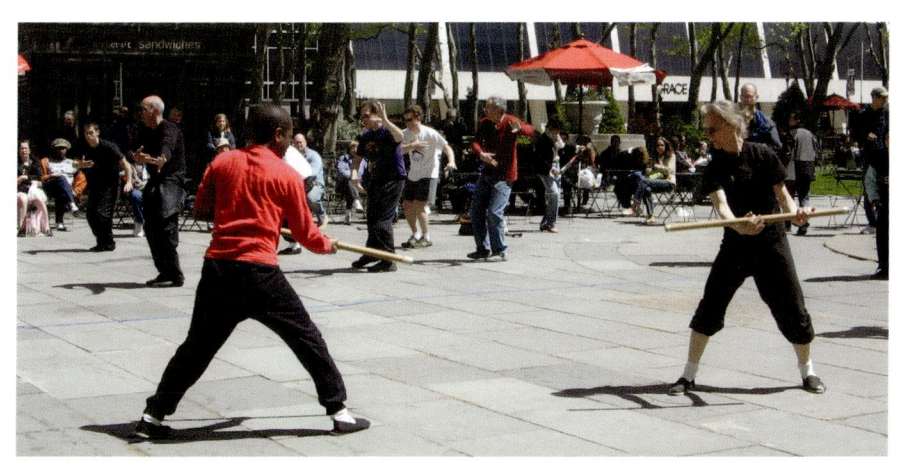

Hyland Harris and Kate Wasilewski demonstrate the Two-person Flute Form.

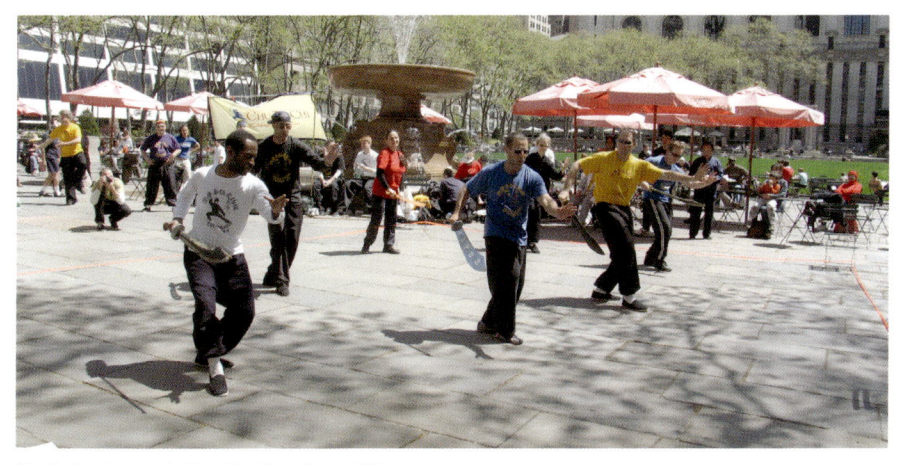

Students demonstrating the Broadsword Form.

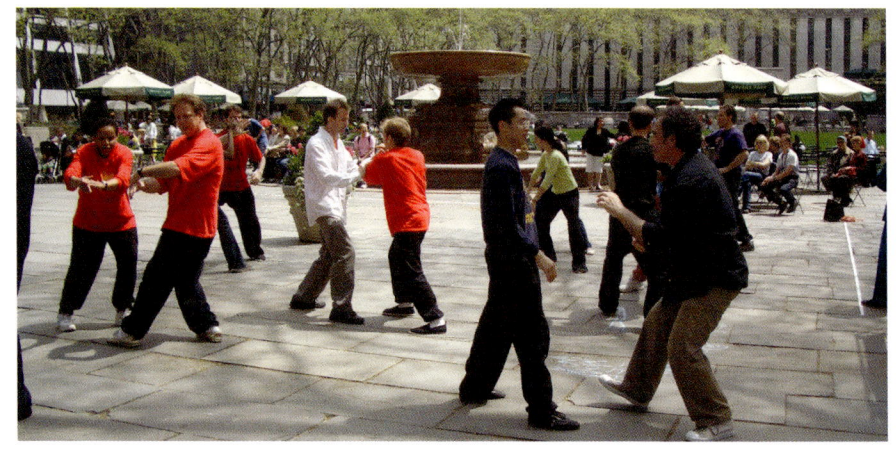

Students doing Push-Hands on World Tai Chi Day in Bryant Park.

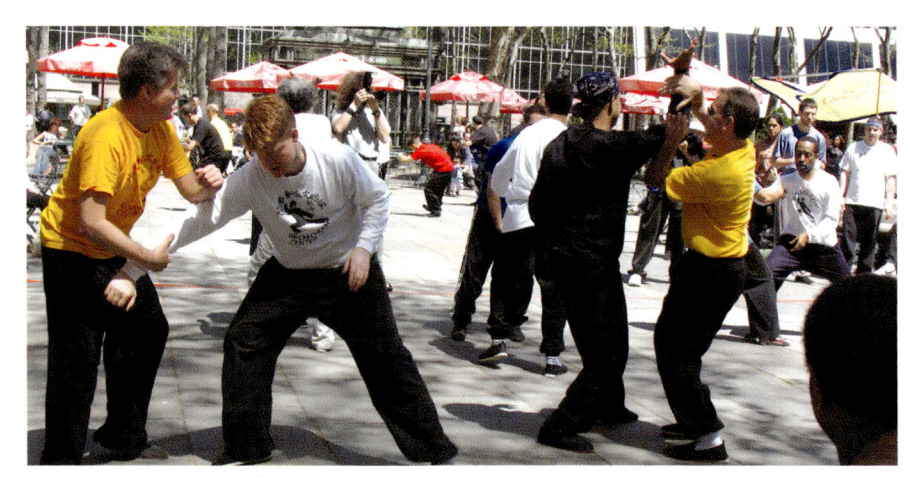

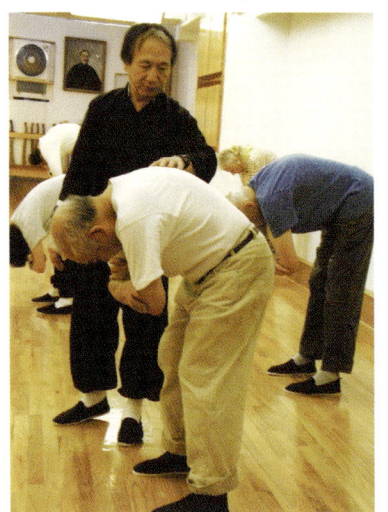

Master Chu helping a student understand the process of aligning his body to fix his back during an Eternal Spring Workshop.

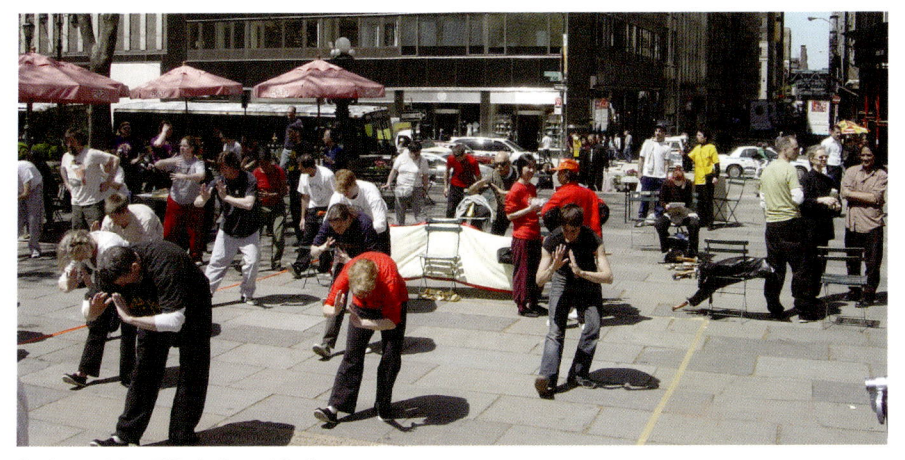

Students doing Pi'Pa in Bryant Park.

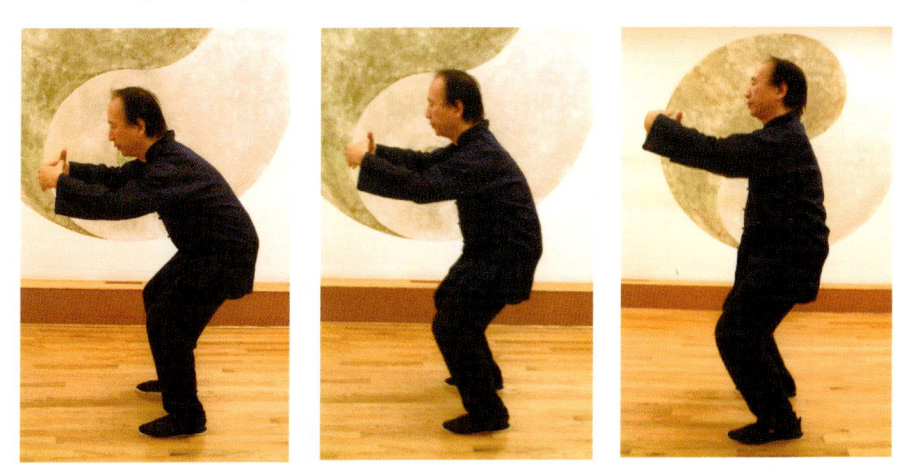

Master Chu demonstrates the way the body angles change depending on an individual's level, see question 6.13.

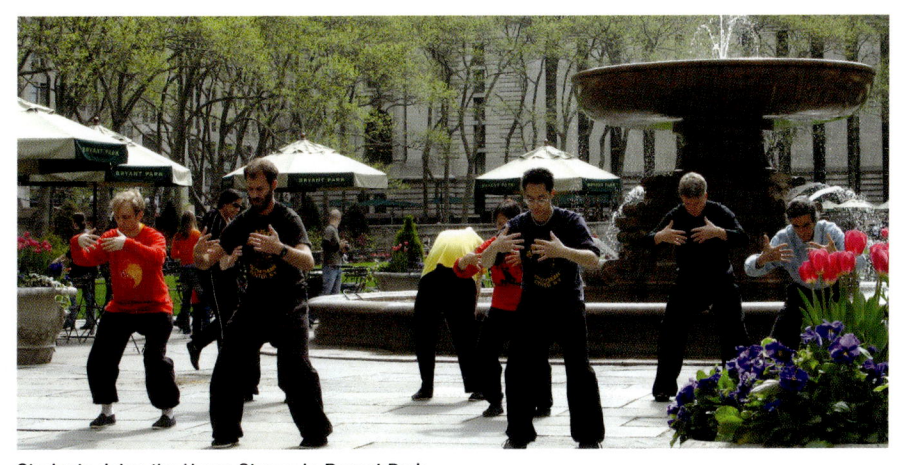

Students doing the Horse Stance in Bryant Park.

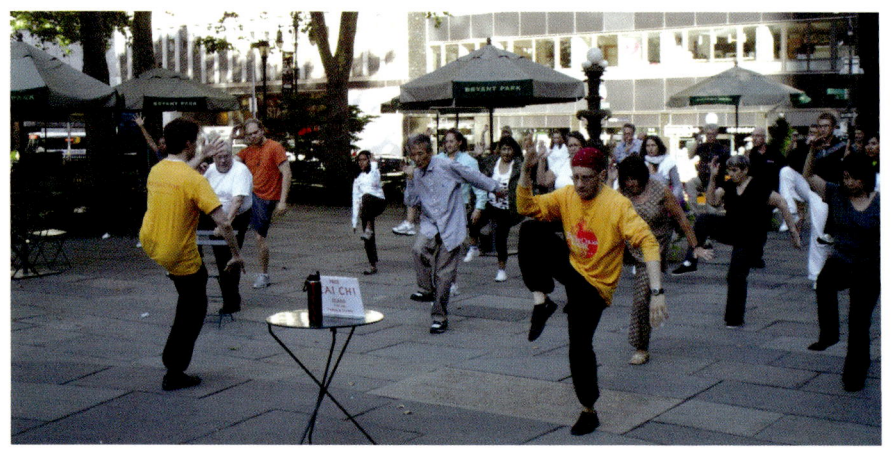

Jeremy W. Hubbell leading Eternal Spring Class in Bryant Park, assisted by Martin Andrews

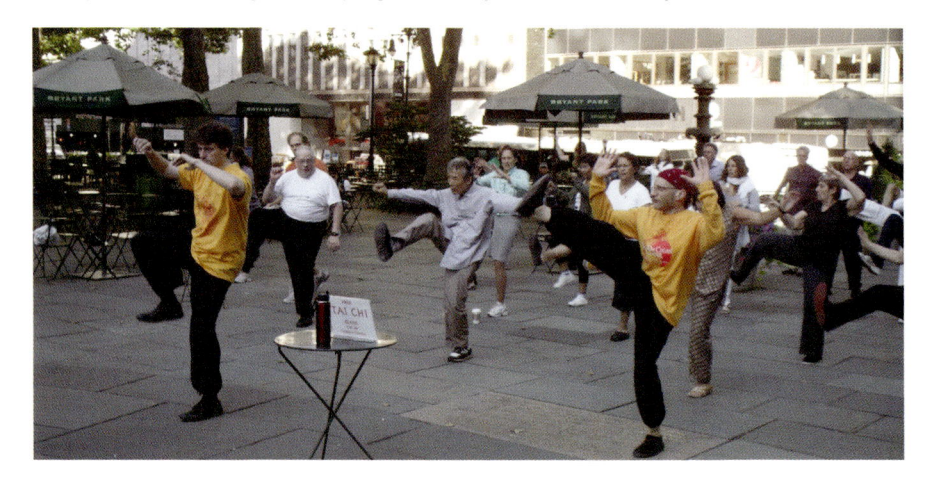

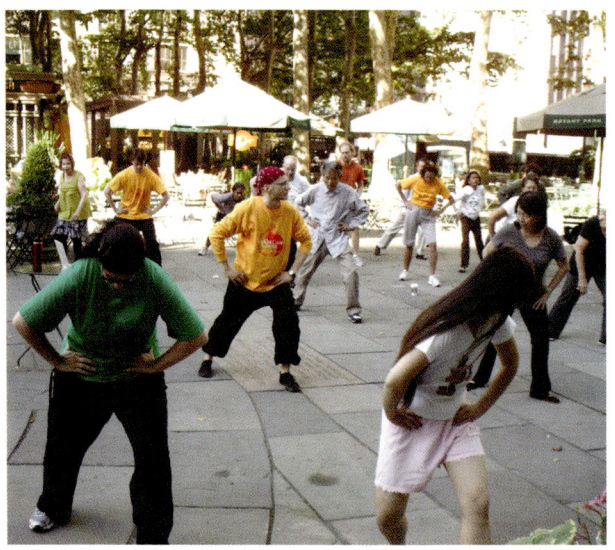

The first picture is Golden Rooster; second is Heel Kick; third picture is Pivoting to Bow Stance.

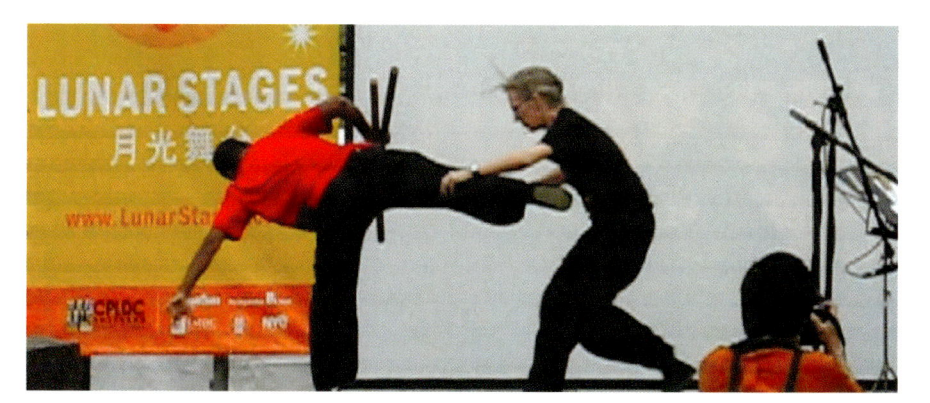

Hyland Harris and Kate Wasilewski demonstrating Two-person Stick on the Lunar Stage in Chinatown.

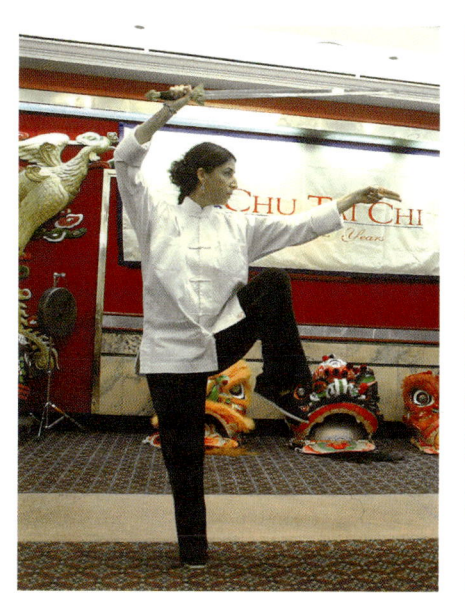

Cynthia Elmas is doing the Double-edged Sword Form at a New Year banquet.

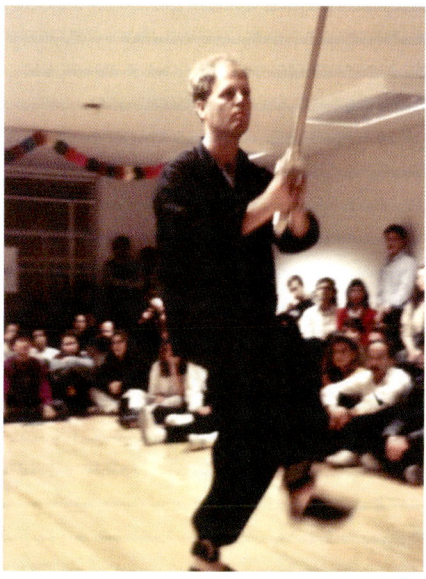

Dick Esterle demonstrating Double-edged Sword at the house-warming party of the Tai Chi Chuan Center.

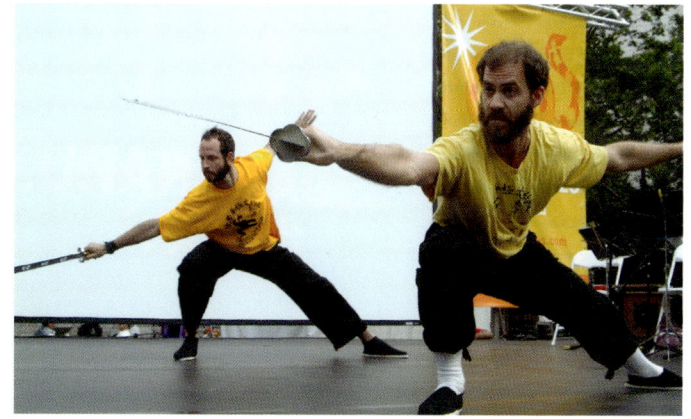

Michael Ballantine and Jesse Shadoan demonstrate the Broadsword Form.

# IV. LEARNING TAI CHI

### 4.1
### Is tai chi for everyone?

The answer is yes, tai chi is good for everyone. However, not too many people are aware of the benefits of tai chi. Also, some people are not willing or ready to learn. Many people have the wrong priorities in life. To me, the highest priorities should be health and self-defense — everything else should be secondary. Tai chi addresses both of these priorities.

### 4.2
### Can I learn tai chi
### from books or videos?

If it were possible, it would require several volumes of books and videos, and a huge amount of patience just to learn the tai chi short form. What a student really needs is a qualified teacher who can provide feedback and corrections. In the beginning, students cannot know if they are making errors. They might use a book or video as a reference to follow the proper sequence of the form, but tai chi is a subtle art which emphasizes balance, focus and root. This makes it difficult for students to learn even when there is a teacher demonstrating right in front of them. Without a teacher's regular feedback and correction, mistakes, missteps and misalignments will be compounded. During training, the tai chi student requires a detailed awareness of specific aspects of body alignment. To begin with, one needs to ensure that the head is suspended, the spine elongated, and the lower back tucked in. It would be impossible for a beginner to gain much of a feel for this from a two-dimensional image.

## 4.3
## What is the correct way of learning the form?

If you want to learn tai chi, it's best to start with some body conditioning, like *Eternal Spring Chi Kung*. Through *Eternal Spring* you work on your breathing and learn proper bodily alignment, both of which are fundamental to tai chi.

After you've done some *Eternal Spring*, you can start taking tai chi classes. In these classes, the focus is on body movement and coordination. Over time, the body becomes flexible and agile. It begins to move as one piece — similar to the way an animal moves. Learning the philosophy and the fighting aspect of tai chi comes later.

I teach the tai chi form one move at a time. This is the traditional way and, in my opinion, the best way. I feel it's best because when you learn one move at a time you can learn to move and align your body correctly. Unfortunately, not many still teach this way. Instead, it has become common to adopt the factory-style approach.

In some factories in China, large groups of workers gather in the morning and follow a teacher as he or she executes the entire form. This way is not really learning. It's just copying and following the movements. Consequently, understanding the movement is poor and few can execute the form without the teacher. This style of learning sacrifices the details of proper body alignment and an internalization of the meaning of the moves. So, they are not actually doing tai chi. Proper body alignment includes doing several things at the same time, such as tucking in the pelvis, staying round, keeping your shoulders down, positioning the knee, balancing, and shifting the weight, which are important to doing each move correctly.

## 4.4
## Please explain the process
## of teaching tai chi one move at a time.

Tai chi is truly a very sophisticated martial art and there is a lot to learn before a person gains a minimum of competence. Therefore, it is best to take it slow. In the first few tai chi classes, you learn to 'tuck in' and keep your hands round as if you are holding a ball. But when you start moving from one move to another it may be difficult to keep your tuck or maintain roundness, and you may look like a mannequin. I call this the first approximation of the form. As time goes by, your hands won't be static like you're holding a ball. They will be smooth. But this takes time. You must learn each move first.

In fact, the way I teach is to break down every move into four or five or six smaller moves. Breaking down the move into smaller steps serves several purposes. Primarily, the move is demystified. If I just say, 'watch and do what I do,' the student may easily get frustrated and go home. Whereas if I say, 'just do these two things for now until I return' the student will memorize those two things. I can then return and add two moves to those two and before the student realizes it, the complex move has been accomplished. By breaking down each move in this manner, the student will practice the form slowly so as to do each of the steps correctly. Practicing slowly, the student begins to reap benefits, such as forgetting the stresses of life through a sustained, focused awareness of the body. Later, teaching correct breathing is easier because the student has already been accustomed to breaking the move down and considering it in sections. While at the beginning nothing particular will be said about fighting, this is the traditional method of teaching tai chi as a martial art.

### 4.5
### Do these smaller parts become one move later on?

Yes. During what I call the second approximation, the smaller parts are linked together. In my school, students begin by learning the entire short form, executing the moves slowly, with a focus on balance, coordination and shifting the weight of the body. After students learn all the moves, they return to the beginning, but now concentrating on corrections. After corrections are finished, students return to the beginning again, now focusing on breathing during each move. Later on, the last step of this learning process takes place when students learn the "fast form." This consists of the same moves as in the short form, but done faster. It is while learning to do the form fast that attention is turned to the fighting application of each move. To be able to learn these applications, it is necessary for you to be able to follow the tai chi principles, like stay tucked in and round from beginning to end of the form. There are many layers to learning the form and there is no sense showing a student how to execute a punch or a kick if he or she can't even remain balanced. Learning the form is training: first to improve the body's flexibility and balance, then to learn how to apply the form in fighting.

### 4.6
### Why am I told to make a ball with my hands
### as I first learn the form?

The process of learning tai chi is not unlike constructing a building; only in this case, the building is you. During each approximation, which is a phase of learning the form, different types of scaffolding and tools are used. Eventually, these will be taken away and your body will be aligned and your form will be correct. To use another analogy, learning the form is like learning to draw. At first, drawing a portrait resembling the subject is nearly impossible. So, one starts by making a face with a sphere and using cylinders for the chest and arms. The result is a pile of shapes, not a portrait. But with time, practice, and guidance from a teacher, the lines of the simple shapes become less pronounced and the person's image becomes recognizable. Holding a ball is a way of gently re-patterning and retraining the body so that the hands do not move independently from the body. This is like putting up a scaffold or using a sphere to draw a face. Gradually, in subsequent approximations, the hands will assume more martial postures and be naturally integrated with the upper body — but the ball is still there. Holding the ball is the first step towards understanding and applying the principle that every time the body moves, the hands should be the ends of a circle composed of the entire upper torso. In addition, holding a ball teaches that the hands correspond with each other — they are not moving separately from each other or the rest of the body.

### 4.7
### What do you mean by 'approximation'? How many approximations are there?

Nobody can execute a skill perfectly the first time. Before you can play a piano well, you must know where the keys are. Likewise, in tai chi, first you have to learn the steps and positions; this is an approximation of the form. As mentioned above, holding a sphere to learn hand and body coordination and keeping the hands immobile are part of this first approximation. Later on, as comfort with the form increases, the student works on not moving the hands at all — this is the second approximation. Since tai chi is a whole body exercise, each approximation involves less moving of individual body parts (like the hands) independently of the whole body, and more moving of the whole body as one piece. In later approximations, the student will be shown how to attend to more detail and, for example, angle the hand in a certain way relative to the rest of the body or the torso relative to the hip and the leg. As when learning to draw a portrait, the student makes a sphere and then learns to make the sphere less pronounced — but the sphere is still there. Likewise, in tai chi, there is a progressive series of refinements whereby the student comes closer to doing the form perfectly, and each stage of a student's progress is an approximation. Tai chi is also like sculpture. To sculpt a block first requires a roughing out of the object intended, then a gradual working of the block with ever more attention to detail until the figure is revealed. Mastering tai chi takes time but by accepting the current condition of one's body, one can approximate the tai chi form and, by doing so, improve the body so as to progress to another approximation. Nobody can do the form perfectly the first time. Learning the form should be approached as a long-term project of training the body wherein you will gradually do it more correctly, with practice and instruction.

### 4.8
### Why am I leaning forward to tuck in? How does this help my alignment and chi flow?

Many people have lower back problems because their bodies are very tight and they cannot tuck in. Consequently, when they bend the knee they arch the back. An arched back is weaker and it blocks the *chi* flow. Through tai chi training, such problems can be fixed by learning to tuck in while doing the form. First, using *Eternal Spring*'s Sleeping Lion exercise, in which the torso leans forward and the legs are kept straight, the lower back is stretched. If this action is done regularly and over time, the lower back loosens up. This is good for the body's alignment and it also makes it easier to tuck in. However, the new ease resulting from the increased flexibility will still not be good enough because you are still weak and the body wants to stick to its old habits. The body wants to be vertical and arch the back again. So, while continuing with conditioning exercises and learning the form, a student can lean forward so as to work on keeping the pelvis tucked in. After a period of training, leaning forward will no longer be necessary.

Tucking in is one of the most important aspects of alignment for internal energy in tai chi because the hip links the upper and lower body together. The hip is the critical point. It affects not only the lower back but the knee as well. The knee should be lined up directly over the toe and you should feel a slight stretch on the outside of the knee (see principle #2 in *The Book of Nei Kung* p. 23, and question 2.8). However, if the back is tight this will not happen and the knee will be stressed. Therefore, so as not to hurt the knee while learning the form, students should lean forward. This makes tucking in easier and makes it possible to move the lower body correctly. In other words, while healing the lower back students lean forward, a kind of scaffolding effect, while the body repairs itself and grows stronger. By leaning forward, the tuck can be maintained and the knee moved correctly.

### 4.9
### When being round, can I just point my shoulders in — why must I concave my chest?

Tucking the pelvis under is the most important aspect of alignment in tai chi. Next comes roundness. Being round means that the upper body is linked together in one piece from the fingertips, through the shoulders to the chest, and down to the *tan tien*. The hands, again, are not separate from the body but are moved by the body's movement. To make the upper body one piece including the hands (so that the hands do not move independently), the chest must be concaved and the back round and lifted. A concaved chest and a round back can open and close together, which moves the arms and hands as parts of the torso. Also, the head must be suspended as if from above. This linkage begins, not in the shoulder, but in the *tan tien* (see question 6.5) Not only does this alignment improve the posture generally, but it makes it possible for the body to deliver effective strikes when fighting. Furthermore, this kind of alignment creates what I call the '*chi vacuum*', an alignment in which the body will create more *chi*. This proper alignment makes for a good posture, which is the basis for good health for daily life or for fighting. Tucking in and staying round improves your posture, your alignment, your *chi* flow, and your health. This is what the tai chi classics meant by "Close the chest and lift the back" (*TCCP&P*, pp. 83, 94). The few points mentioned here are essential to doing tai chi: if you are not doing them, you are not doing real tai chi. To do tai chi, the hand and body move together, you are tucked in, the head is suspended, the chest is concave, and the back is round.

## 4.10
### How can I suspend my head while leaning forward, concave my chest, and do the move — isn't this too much to do at the same time?

Although it seems like a lot, in fact all of these things are necessary for correct alignment. The head should be properly placed relative to the body while linking the body parts together into one piece. Successful movement while in proper alignment produces maximum *chi* for the effort spent, while at the same time healing the body. Learning to move the body correctly is difficult at first. For this reason, practice slowly and concentrate on one aspect of alignment at a time while doing one movement at a time. First, concentrate on tucking in. As you grow accustomed to tucking in, be aware of the other principles of alignment: work on concaving the chest and lifting the back second, work on head suspended third. Doing each movement slowly will teach the body to move correctly and make correct movement second nature. Eventually, the body will tuck in all the time and you can concentrate on the next aspect of alignment, like concave chest. To improve the body, do not do tai chi as if it is a series of steps to complete; instead do each movement as a self-massage, a self-alignment adjustment. If you do tai chi from this perspective, you will progress towards doing tai chi more correctly. The closer you get to doing the moves correctly (reflecting the tai chi principles) the more benefit you will experience. The time invested in tai chi is time invested in your health. Do the best you can — progress comes with patience, diligence and perseverance.

## 4.11
### In simple terms, please list the basic tai chi principles a beginner should keep in mind.

Always follow these tai chi principles:
> *The lower back should be straight, never arched.*
> *The knees should be positioned over the toes.*
> *The head should face the hands with the eyes looking past the hands.*
> *The form should be smooth and continuous without hesitation at the same height, with all movements executed at the same speed.*
> *Movement should always come from the* tan tien.
> *One should not bounce up and down or move any part of the body independently of the rest.*
> *The shoulders should always be dropped, so as to maintain a connection with the arms.*
> *The body should always be rounded, not angular.*
> *Breathing should be through the nose down to the* tan tien: *long, deep, small, and smooth.*

## 4.12
## You mention alignment all the time.
## Why is alignment so important in tai chi?

At all times — whether the body is static or dynamic — it should be balanced and coordinated. For this to happen, the body must be aligned correctly. For example, if a building is not aligned properly it tilts to one side. This incorrect center of gravity creates stress on the rest of the building, making it likely to topple over. The same is true of the human body. If it is not aligned correctly, the body's center of gravity will be unstable and all the available strength will need to be used for balance.

The position of the knee is important in bodily alignment. It does not matter if you are standing still or doing something requiring the knee to bend — the knee should always be in the right place. The knee should be pointed slightly outward: knee over toe. In *The Book of Nei Kung*, I illustrate this point (p. 23). Also, arching the lower back puts the knee in the wrong place, which diminishes the health benefit of tai chi and may cause injury. This is incorrect alignment. This is a common mistake for many tai chi practitioners around the world. Correct alignment gives you rooting and the flexibility to move. Anybody who ignores their alignment is just moving around and will never get anything close to true tai chi, let alone a higher level.

## 4.13
## What are corrections? Why do people who have
## been doing tai chi for a long time and even teaching
## tai chi still come to class for corrections?

It is human nature to want to do things well. Look at the record of human effort in the arts and sciences of humans as shown in museums — thousands of people over thousands of years striving to perfect portraiture or scientific understanding. Tai chi is both an art and a science in that it has principles that must be followed, it must be practiced regularly to flourish and grow, and it takes forever to perfect but the pursuit is enjoyable. Take mathematics. First you do arithmetic, then algebra, geometry, trigonometry, analytical geometry, calculus, differential equations and so on. At each level you can solve a problem with ever-greater sophistication. Similarly, you first learn to write simple sentences with a subject, verb, and object. In time you can use participles, modifiers, and pronouns. Continuing, you can write poetry, prose, essays, and the like. In these examples, progress depends on acquiring skill, often with help from a teacher or books, and then practicing that skill until you are ready for something more complicated. There is no end to the pursuit of perfection.

It is the same with tai chi. Through practice over time, the body and mind improve, becoming more integrated and, therefore, able to do tai chi can more correctly. Tai chi is a martial art and to apply the moves correctly, the body must be able to move in one piece, but it takes time for the body to be able to do this. Tai chi is different from linear exercises. A push-up is a push-up is a push-up. But tai chi is not always the same and it is hard to know what to do by yourself, especially when your body has adapted to one approximation and is ready to learn another. Then, you must consult a teacher.

By way of analogy, think of the archer. Archery has just one movement: draw the bow and shoot the arrow. But through body and mind connection, correct alignment, and a feeling for the bow, the archer becomes more accurate and more deadly. This takes time. Archery is easy to teach in one hour, but a dedicated archer will shoot differently after 10 years of practice. To be in the imperial guard, like my great uncle, you had to be able to ride a galloping horse and hit a coin 100 yards away. To do that takes great skill and many years of practice. Tai chi is like that: practice and constant correction leads to improvement. In archery, you want to hit the target with great frequency and from far away. Your next goal is to improve your speed of execution and your stability, whether you are standing still or on a galloping horse. Finally, you graduate from a weak bow to a strong bow. Each gradation of difficulty requires correct alignment and mind-body coordination. It takes years to train these things, and archery has just one move. Tai chi has many facets of training. Push-hands takes years to develop until, by just a touch of the opponent's hands, you know his weakness. In fighting, you develop more speed and the ability to put more pounds of force behind your punch. These gradations of development require a lot of adjustment and correction. It is almost impossible to do this on your own: even professional tennis players need coaches, especially when they are number one in the world. In the old days, tai chi masters could fight 100 armed opponents at once and beat them. These masters needed someone to help them adjust their form since no matter how good someone is at a skill, he cannot see himself.

Progress in the form should also include developing related skills, such as push-hands. Then you can learn to fight one opponent: then multiple opponents. Then you can learn the weapons forms. So the levels go on and on, and it is up to you how far you will progress. But to gain the correct form and move the body in one piece, you need feedback from a teacher. I call getting that feedback "corrections." Corrections can be done during any tai chi class at my school. Just as education begins with grade school and continues through graduate school, so learning tai chi begins with first approximations and continues through to corrections. Without a good solid foundation, you cannot proceed to a higher level of understanding and execution. There are no shortcuts.

### 4.14
### Do corrections ever end?

Tai chi is both an art and a science; it is an expression of beauty based on a set of principles. Mastery is the lifetime pursuit of perfection of tai chi. In the beginning, you need assistance from a teacher in learning the form. Then, you need a teacher to correct you until you can correct yourself. After learning the form, the teacher reminds you verbally and may, by helping you do the movements, physically aid you in doing the movements better. If you are genuine in your pursuit of tai chi, then you are always a student. If you are lucky, you will always receive feedback from a knowledgeable teacher; but if eventually you find yourself on your own, you can continue to improve daily by staying true to the tai chi principles. Even Yang Cheng-fu felt he was still improving his form up to the end of his life. His form changed as his body changed over his lifetime pursuit of mastery of the tai chi principles. In time, his body became more loose, strong, round, relaxed, and rooted. Developing a tai chi body takes time. People have spent a long time arguing about whether doing tai chi as Yang did it early in life or late in life is better. I think this debate is a waste of time. You cannot imitate Yang Cheng-fu because you are not him; you can only admire his mastery, which reflects a lifetime of correct practice. Each person has to do tai chi according to the tai chi principles, and what that means for a person just beginning tai chi will be different from what that means for that person after 50 years of practicing correctly. Tai chi is an art, with a set of movements to be done, but it is also a process of training the body. In this pursuit, our understanding of the art becomes deeper and deeper. So, corrections by a teacher may end but improvement never ends.

### 4.15
### What, specifically, is the best path to progress?

First, when practicing, try to do everything as correctly as possible by understanding and applying the principles throughout the form. This requires discipline, mindfulness, and going slowly. Don't just do the form as an exercise to get through, like doing 10 push-ups in the morning. Keeping in mind the principles, do the form as an expression of the art and science of tai chi. It is a bit like trying to draw a perfect circle in one shot. You can never do it, but by practicing every day you can get closer and closer. In the same way, try to follow the principles as you do the form. You can never do it perfectly, but you will get closer and closer as you get better and better. Meanwhile, you will reap the benefits of improved health.

Next, apply concrete measurement to your practice. Use a watch to time yourself to see how slowly you can go, and then go even more slowly. If you are becoming adept at applying the principles and going slowly, focus on correct breathing and alignment. This is where learning *chi kung* helps. Use the focused breathing principles you learn in *chi kung* class to breathe during the form. Then, time yourself to see how fast you can go — the faster the better. Do not skip anything and do not compromise any principle.

The next step is to work on distinguishing between hardness and softness. When striking, intend to strike with power; when yielding, intend to yield with softness. That is how you pursue improvement: establish a measure of where you are and then work to move beyond that point. Have a goal to work on while doing the form each and every time, so you don't just go through the motions. A good teacher will guide you in this process.

It is possible to do this on your own provided you have a good foundation in the art. However, working completely on your own is more difficult. If you are on your own, you will have to remind yourself constantly to tuck in, stay round, and be rooted.

This art is very challenging, but the rewards are great. Your body is constantly developing, like a growing tree. Tai chi helps the body develop by enabling it to have a healthier root and trunk. As you pursue perfection in tai chi, your body will change in amazing ways. For this to happen, you will need self-discipline, mindfulness, and consistency (see *TCCP&P*, p. 68). As *"The Song of the Thirteen Movements"* says, "you are practicing tai chi… for a prolonged life — like an eternal spring" (*TCCP&P*, p. 91).

### 4.16
### How do you learn the most from a teacher?

Any school follows a curriculum. Once you find a reputable school and teacher, follow the curriculum the best you can. Approach the teacher with faith and believe that his or her reputation is well earned and it is based on the curriculum taught. Don't question every single thing you are taught. If you knew tai chi, you would not be seeking a teacher so do not pretend to know more than the teacher you sought out for instruction. Having faith in a teacher does not mean having blind or religious faith. Rather, you ought to trust that you are on the right path and this teacher can lead you for now. If you have doubts, ask questions, but you must be sincere. Don't ask a question just to embarrass or trip up a teacher — is that why you sought out the teacher? Instead, stick with the teacher, for it is a common experience that when you are ready to learn, the teacher for you will soon appear. If you are not ready to learn, then even if the greatest teacher of all stood before you and taught you the correct answer 1,000 times, you still would not learn it.

Learning is a process you must go through and that process is unique to each individual. The process is also different depending on the subject. Learning math is different from learning tai chi. For tai chi, less talk, more practice, is best. In fact, the *Tao Te Ching* mentions the importance of "teaching without words," teaching by example and also learning by doing (see chapter 2). Practice and you will discover certain points by yourself, which you can then confirm with a teacher. The first few years of learning a new discipline are as crucial as the early stages of plant growth. First, the soil must be prepared and the seed, say, of a tree properly planted. Then the seedling must be protected for a time. Soon enough, the tree will be able to grow by itself for hundreds of years — long past the time of the person who planted the seed. With a good foundation, you too can grow strong by yourself. A good tai chi foundation requires a few years for thorough understanding. Don't forget, it takes just a half a year to learn the form, then another year to learn push-hands and fighting. So, 3-5 years is still the beginning period. That period is critical to ensuring future success. You will benefit right from the beginning but you have to allow time to obtain a strong foundation.

A good teacher will teach you what you are ready to learn. Many students look for a shortcut. They always want to go to the next move even though they are not proficient in the technique they are currently learning. What they don't know is that a good curriculum is already the "shortcut." It will take them on the shortest path to their goal. Of course, even with the correct guidance, students must practice on their own. For example, when I show a student a punch, the student must practice it thousands of times. The punch must become so natural it is second nature. That way, when the time comes to use it, it will be automatic.

### 4.17
### Can you give another example of following curriculum?

A student's father came to my school and told me his son wanted to learn fighting, but did not want to learn any "esoteric philosophy behind it." First of all, the philosophy that underlies tai chi, which is Taoism, is not esoteric. It's very practical. Secondly, fighting is not just fighting. It's not just my technique versus yours.

Fighting is more than meets the eye. It includes studying a philosophy of life. It would be ridiculous to expect to become a great fighter just by punching and kicking. Both the body and mind must be powerful. The power comes from a strong foundation. The foundation for my students consists of five pillars: *nei kung*, *chi kung*, tai chi form, meditation, and Taoist philosophy and the Taoist stages of self-cultivation (see chapter 7).

Tai chi is a material science in that we train to fight and study the techniques of fighting, sweat and hit. Training *nei kung* makes the body strong so that, being hit by an opponent, is not an automatic injury and it might not even hurt at all. *Nei kung* also builds rootedness. The tai chi form trains balance, agility and movements for self-defense application. *Chi kung* develops your diaphragm breathing and body alignment. Later, students take Fight Class where they drill certain moves to make them second nature. Meditation and Taoist study give you mental clarity and a philosophy of life that will guide all your actions. Taoist cultivation is a science of human interactions, relationships, and the dynamics of society. As a soft science, we study ethics, morality, and the way things actually are. Studying the Tao is to study how nature actually is, not what religion or politic parties say. Through this type of training, you develop a calm mind that is able to grasp the nature of any situation as it really is, so you can handle an attack, mental or physical, from any direction. All of these components are necessary to make you a competent or high-level fighter.

Students (or their parents) do not have enough knowledge to make their own curriculum. In the same way, you wouldn't ask a college freshman to write a degree curriculum.

### 4.18
### Do some students take a long time
### to learn the form?

The answer is yes. I had one student whose body alignment was in bad shape. She was arching her back instead of tucking in her pelvis, and her knee positioning was a problem. I could not teach her tai chi until I helped her fix her alignment.

It took over 10 classes to teach her the first move. She gave up at first because it was difficult. A few weeks later she returned, determined to finish and eventually she completed the entire form. The benefit starts right from the beginning but every student learns at a different speed.

### 4.19
### Do some students learn the form faster than others?

Yes. Some students pick up the form quickly. However, a student who learns quickly might not feel like practicing. He might think that he already "knows the move." But it is through regular and correct practice that you get the benefits of tai chi.

In fact, the more you practice the form, the more benefits you get. Doing the form twice in a row is better than doing it only once. Doing the form three times is better than doing it twice.

Through practicing, you tune up the body and make the energy go deeper and deeper. Simply knowing a move or even the entire form is not enough.

### 4.20
### So what would be an ideal student?

An ideal student picks up the form easily, enjoys it, and understands the importance of practice. He or she sets personal goals and works to meet those goals. The ideal student would do this for all aspects of training.

A student should be serious, inquisitive, and desirous of learning. He or she must also have the ability and time to do the requisite practice; she must do the work and always seek to move forward in her understanding and ability to do tai chi. In Chinese there is a saying about the ideal student being someone who can figure out the four corners of a table by being shown only one corner. In other words, a good student does not need to be told everything. Rather, if a principle is conveyed clearly and understood, it can be applied to different problems and situations. Since to master tai chi is first to master and mold your own body, the ideal student must also be willing and able to studiously mold his or her own body and welcome mental and physical changes that come with that work.

In addition to his or her own study, the ideal student helps other students. This generosity helps the teacher and the school. By being a constructive part of the school, she improves her own understanding while helping others to advance too. In Taoism, it is taught that all are equal. According to this view, students should have humility and not be interested in rank or prestige, only in improvement of the ability to do tai chi. Tai chi is an internal art and each person strives to do the art to the best of her ability. Along with this comes the idea of *wu wei*. The ideal student does not struggle but lets the process of learning, understanding, and improvement happen in time.

The ideal tai chi student loves the art of tai chi and is immersed in it. Such a student does tai chi for the sake of doing it — not for personal glory or gain.

Her distinction will come when others recognize her correct understanding and application of the tai chi principles. The ideal student will distinguish herself from others and will be a good teacher and promoter of the art in the future.

### 4.21
### Why is it so important to be a good student?

The art of tai chi is very beautiful. Only by immersing yourself in it and always striving to make your practice better and better can you fully enjoy the art. To me, this art is like a Chinese treasure and it shouldn't be wasted. Wasting tai chi is to not do it — just leave the principles and forms in books. It is truly a treasure that gets better in time but only by careful adherence and diligent practice of the principles that others have already discovered. It is not up to us to invent tai chi, only to practice it correctly. If that is done, the art improves and so does your body.

I often say that tai chi is a science. Well, science advances by building on the past or, as is commonly said, by standing on the shoulders of giants: Einstein stands on the shoulders of Newton who stands on the shoulders of Galileo. Each is humble before the past and before science as a whole. Likewise, today's practitioners of tai chi stand on the shoulders of past practitioners to carry on improving and polishing the treasure that is tai chi.

### 4.22
### What's the best way to motivate myself to reach a higher-level in tai chi and *nei kung*?

A guitarist can play guitar for 30 years without improving his technique. The same is true of tai chi. It's possible to coast for years and not get to a higher level. You need challenges to push yourself. If a guitarist has an upcoming concert, he'll work harder to prepare. For tai chi, you can vigorously prepare to enter a tournament. This will motivate you and make you train.

I learned how to play the harmonica when I was in elementary school. I can still pick it up and play any song by ear, but that doesn't mean I'm as good as someone who has been studying and working on technique for 50 years. I'm still a novice.

Learning the mechanics of the tai chi form doesn't mean you really know tai chi or self-defense. You must attend to detail and push yourself. This takes effort, but if you enjoy the art, it is not hard work. Anything you enjoy doing is not hard work.

### 4.23
### How does one judge his progress in tai chi, *nei kung* and meditation?

When a student first learns tai chi, he does what I call first approximations: the frame, the structure, tucking in, concaving the chest, roundness, moving from the *tan tien*, etc. Later after a period of practice, the student should take corrections, working on details to refine the execution of the movements and get closer to real tai chi. I suggest all students take correction classes periodically. There are many levels of refinement in tai chi. The more corrections one gets, the more progress one will see.

One's progress in tai chi can also be measured quantitatively. The more proficient one is, the slower and then the faster one can do the form. Therefore, a student can time the form to measure progress. Do the form slow, meditatively and correctly, taking 15 minutes to finish, for example. Then, aim to stretch it to 20 minutes or so. On the other end, try to do the form as fast as possible (still observing tai chi principles). One has to be very good to do the form in one minute, for example. It is an important part of practice to keep track of where you are in this way. Work on both ends of the speed spectrum in the form.

However, it is important not to compromise the correctness of the form even though the clock is running. It does not serve the purpose of training to do the form in a sloppy manner just for the speed. To do so is to fool yourself about the actual progress being made.

With *nei kung*, too, a student needs corrections to continue refining the form. To determine one's progress, time how long you can hold the Horse Stance, Playing P'i P'a, and so on. Pay attention to your level of relaxation while doing these stances. The goal is to hold the posture for a long time while being relaxed — a good Playing P'i Pa held for 10 minutes should be easy, not a great struggle. Similarly, use a stopwatch to see how long you can sit in meditation.

Finally, a good way to measure progress is to take a test. I offer tests in tai chi and *nei kung* leading to certification. Test preparation provides an incentive to stay focused during practice and to come to class for corrections on ever more precise details. This way, one can greatly improve one's form. Without a test, a student can become complacent and remain on the same level for a long time. It is the same with any art. When a concert or an exhibition is coming up, an artist will be more motivated to put in the work necessary for a successful performance.

### 4.24
### After the Short Form, are there other forms to learn?

Yes, one should do the long form. Some martial art systems offer 30 or 40 different forms that a student can learn in just a few years. In addition, these forms typically last for only a few minutes or less. In the tai chi long form, all the elementary and advanced moves are compiled into one continuous, congruent form of 108 movements that takes 35 to 40 minutes to do. The practice requires a student to aim to perfect the one form by repetition. Due to the style of the practice, the system has been preserved for over 800 years with minimal changes. Tai chi is sometimes called the "Long Fist", just as the Yangtse River is called the "Long River". It is called the "Long Fist" because one does the form for a long duration of time and, like a long river that keeps flowing, never ceasing, one does the movements without break (*TCCP&P*, p. 64). After learning the long form, one should keep taking corrections that will add more detail and depth to one's practice. After learning the long form, one can learn the *San Shou* (a two-person empty-hand form) and weapons forms.

### 4.25
### Why breathe in when striking, both in the form and when fighting?

Tai chi is the study of the natural function of the body as well as a method of training that follows the natural operations of the body. When a person uses strength, the breath is held involuntarily. Try pushing a heavy object. What did you do? First, you touched the object with the hands to sense the weight, then, hands still touching it, your butt moved back and your legs got behind it so that your pelvis tucked in as your body lowered to, as they say, 'get behind it.' Once set, you breathed in as the push was engaged. The breath was then held as the push lasted, and then, when it was over, the breath was released. In other words, when you use strength, you must breathe in and hold the breath. You cannot exert a lot of strength if you breathe out while using strength.

In a fighting situation, you breathe in when you want to strike, then while you are striking you are holding your breath for however long you are in contact with the opponent. When the strike is finished and your body is out of contact with the opponent, you breathe out. In this context, think of the body as a tire. To make the tire as firm and strong as possible to support a car, it must be full of air. So the valve must take in air to make the tire its strongest and then close to hold the air while the car is to be supported. Once it is no longer necessary to support the car, the valve can open and let the air out — relaxing the tire. Likewise, when you are striking, you want to be as strong and firm as you can be, so you fill up with air. Then, after punching, you breathe out so you can breathe in again to be strong for the next punch. Chen Wei-ming says, "when you breathe in, you are naturally lifted up and at the same time able to lift your opponent up" (*TCCP&P*, pp. 138-139).

There are many misconceptions about breathing. Many people, perhaps most, learn this backwards. They learn to make noises or breathe out while striking. This may have arisen in recent times because of the obvious lack of real battle experience (changes in warfare have minimized the need for professional soldiers who know hand-to-hand combat, though soldiers still learn these skills). But the other reason has to do with misunderstanding the timing and purpose of breathing out. If you have ever tried to move something too heavy for you and the only result was a strained noise from your mouth, you know that noise is easily produced after such effort. Some people assume the noise is made while executing the power. In fact, the noise comes from the exhale *after* the strike. You can experiment with this yourself by breathing out while you use strength and you will see that your power is reduced. When you strike, the object will strike back — this is basic physics, action/reaction.

So you must be as solid as possible to not only strike the opponent but to withstand the reaction of the opponent to being hit so you can follow through with your strike. You can only do that by breathing in and holding the breath. Once you have finished the strike, breathe out.

# V. PRACTICING TAI CHI

### 5.1
### It seems that tai chi does not emphasize discipline to the degree that other systems do.

Some schools rely heavily on external discipline: the teacher drills his students like a master sergeant drills his soldiers. The orders come from outside, and above. In tai chi, the discipline must come from within. This makes it much more difficult. Nobody tells you what to do. You have to make decisions for yourself. It is like learning to play music. When learning an instrument, a student must enjoy it, but playing music also takes discipline if the student is going to attain a level above a recreational musician. Likewise, daily tai chi practice concentrating on perfecting the movements is the only way to reach a high level. One reason some people who begin to learn tai chi do not stay the course is that they lack internal discipline, whether for practicing tai chi, a musical instrument, or other things. However, it is not only a matter of discipline to learn tai chi but an openness and ability to understand a whole system of health and a way of thinking as well. By understanding the complete meaning of tai chi, it is easier to develop and sustain discipline and enthusiasm for daily practice. Therefore, forceful, external discipline is not only not required but counterproductive. Students who achieve success in tai chi become well-centered, self-disciplined individuals, because they become their own master.

### 5.2
### Should there be any pain when practicing tai chi?

As in any serious exercise there will be some level of discomfort in the muscles, tendons and joints: that is how the body becomes stronger and it is to be expected. It is, however, important to distinguish the normal pain of working out from pain that indicates damage is being caused. In tai chi, many people experience slight back pain when they first start practicing. If a student follows my instructions correctly, yet the pain continues, it means there are some problems with the back. Here, pain is a signal that the body is adjusting itself to a correct posture by straightening the back. It is a good sign.

Generally speaking, pain in any part of the body is fine — except the knee. Pain in the outer muscles around the knee is OK. However, pain felt inside the kneecap indicates incorrect alignment. It means the pelvis is not tucked in and the body weight is falling in the wrong place. Even when walking up and down stairs, the knees will be free of stress if the pelvis is tucked in and the torso leans forward to maintain correct alignment.

If you follow the guideline for correct body alignment described in *The Book of Nei Kung* — knees out, tuck in, etc. — the body should fall into a correct posture. Difficulty holding correct posture is a sign of some kind of injury in the body. Every time correct alignment is held, there will be a slight pain. This is correct pain and a sign of healing. Obviously, however, too much pain is not good. It indicates that the injury is severe. In this case, stop what you are doing, back off, and pace yourself.

As we train, the muscles and tendons become stronger; however, this is a slow process. As the body ages, it takes longer to heal. Therefore, the saying "no pain, no gain" is correct. Or, as I say, "correct pain, much gain."

## 5.3
## Why lean forward and round the back?
## I thought the back should be straight and vertical in Tai Chi?

When a person stands up straight, the body has a natural curve. Some people have more of a curve than others. Bending the knees without tucking in will align the hips and pelvis incorrectly and this incorrect alignment will put pressure on the knees. Plus, without tucking in, the lower back will freeze and be unable to twist independently of the hips. A fundamental tai chi principle is 'the waist is like an axle' — it must be free to move (*TCCP&P,* p. 82). So, to follow tai chi principles and utilize the body's full function, you must tuck the pelvis under. If you do this, you will avoid fusing the hips and lower back together. Also, by tucking in, the hips align properly with the knees and the knees can be angled correctly. This will allow the feet to be firmly planted on the ground, forming a solid root. Tucking in allows your back to be straight. The principle of the straight back does not mean a linear straightness like on a machine, but rather as if the back is a string of beads suspended from the top of the head and each bead can twist.

Beginners have problems tucking in the pelvis. Their back is stiff because they are too sedentary. By leaning forward while undertaking the tai chi form, the torso is free to move without affecting the hips, and the pressure on the knees is reduced.

Leaning forward is necessary for 80-90% of beginning students. This is good for the lower back and good for the knees (see *The Book of Nei Kung* p. 23).

### 5.4
### Are there other reasons why we should lean forward?

Another reason to lean forward is for attack. You can see this clearly in photographs of old masters like Yang Cheng-fu, Tung Ying-chieh, and Dong Hu Ling. They all tuck in and lean forward. The forward-leaning posture adds to their striking power. Tai chi is a martial art, and it's correct to lean forward in attacking movements.

### 5.5
### Do we also lean back?

Yes, leaning back is one component of yielding. When a strong wind blows, a rigid tree may break, whereas the tall grass will simply yield to the force of the wind and bend in whichever direction it blows. In tai chi self-defense, the same rule applies. When your opponent attacks, bend back like the grass with a strong root in the ground. When his attacking power is finished, spring back up and lean forward to counterattack. For instance, if someone throws a punch toward my head, I adjust my footwork, shift, twist, and lean back just enough to get away from his attack. At the same time I stick to his arm until his power is finished. Continuing to stick, I then prepare to strike. Finally, I lean forward and attack him with my palm using Brush Knee and Twist Step.

### 5.6
### What is the importance of smoothness in practicing tai chi?

I would say that smoothness is essential, and that slowness will bring smoothness. When tai chi movements are done correctly, the body operates like a whip. Any stiffness along the length of the whip will disrupt its smooth, wave-like motion. If the tai chi movements are not done smoothly, the flow of *chi* in the body will be disrupted. Proper attention and practice allow us to find and eliminate these breaks in the body's movement and in the *chi* flow.

After all, everyone has some tightness in his or her body, and this becomes more common with age. Without exercise, the body and the joints are not nourished by a regular *chi* flow. As a result, stiffness and arthritis can result. Practicing tai chi slowly and smoothly can have an immediate healing effect on joint problems because, when done correctly, all parts of the body have a chance to open and heal.

## 5.7
## We learn the tai chi form very meticulously. How do we bridge the gap between including all the details of the form and achieving smoothness?

Yes, the form must be learned systematically. In order to teach tai chi, I have broken down each move of the form into several sections and enumerated them. Students practice one section at a time and connect them in a sequence to make one correct move. Later, especially when learning the fast form, focus turns to connecting all sections smoothly without stopping. Training correctly involves meticulous attention and adherence to the basic principles at each point in the form. The whole body must move from the *tan tien* as one unit.

This makes tai chi a very challenging exercise. It is the art of moving the body naturally — relaxed, comfortable, and without unnecessary stress. When the moves are done right, energy moves noticeably like waves originating from the center (the *tan tien* see question 6.5) to the extremities of the body. Such a feeling indicates you are doing the moves correctly. In addition, correct tai chi enables movement with such rootedness and balance that yielding requires minimal effort while attacks are done with tremendous force.

Again, to achieve smoothness in the form, pay attention to the details — the "tai chi-ness" — in each section of each move. The head should be suspended, pelvis tucked in, knees out, chest concave; the movement should be from the *tan tien*; the eyes should follow the action, and so on. In my DVD on the tai chi short form, there is a list of at least 15 important points to follow. Work toward achieving all of them throughout the form by focusing on one move at a time, for each move is different and presents a different set of challenges.

## 5.8
## How do you coordinate breathing to slow movement in tai chi?

When doing tai chi slowly, breathing also becomes slow. The body's movement ultimately coordinates naturally with the breathing. Each tai chi movement involves an "opening and closing" of the body as one connected unit. The arms and legs do not move independently but, rather, move along with the rest of the body. Ultimately, moving slowly helps to unite the body, the mind and the breath. This integration occurs naturally with consistent practice over time.

## 5.9
## Can the slow movement of tai chi benefit the cardiovascular system?

Yes, it can. Most beginners who practice tai chi slowly, immediately notice that their heart rate increases and their breathing becomes heavier. This indicates that the cardiovascular system is being exercised. The deep breathing in tai chi (whether done slowly or quickly) heals and strengthens the cardiovascular system. Eventually, with correct practice, the heart rate will remain relatively low even when you execute fast movements.

## 5.10
## In what way does slow movement benefit the cardiovascular system?

Slow movement is more beneficial to the system than fast movement. When moving slowly, the heart and the muscles surrounding it expand and contract naturally. Gradually, they build the strength to handle faster movement. Engaging in fast-paced exercise with sudden and quick movements before the body is ready can damage the heart. This is exactly how athletes injure themselves — undue emotional and physical stress on their hearts causes heart attacks. In tai chi, practicing slow movements expands and contracts every part of the body smoothly. As the heart becomes stronger, one can practice the same movement faster.

One point that I always emphasize to my students is relaxation. Relaxation means being calm and at ease, flexible, alert, and without unnecessary tension. It does not mean being limp and inattentive as if daydreaming. The body needs to be in a relaxed state to function most efficiently. When it is not relaxed, the entire system is needlessly taxed, which can damage the body. For example, running fast is fine with careful self-monitoring. If the breathing gets too heavy or the heart starts to beat too fast, then stop. A machine is not required for this monitoring: just pay attention to how you feel. There is little gain in forcing exercise — you will only injure yourself.

By practicing tai chi, one develops a healthier, stronger heart. Health of both body and mind is indispensable to any kind of martial art practice. People often associate kung fu with aggression, but it is actually the opposite. A good fighter needs to have a calm and relaxed mind so as to make a quick and accurate judgment of a situation and defend as necessary. Strengthening the cardiovascular system is merely one aspect of tai chi training. In order to achieve the most benefit, a student needs to train not only slowly but also correctly.

## 5.11
## What is continuous form?

"Continuous Form" refers to executing a tai chi form a number of times in succession. The more times you can repeat the form and the longer you spend doing the tai chi forms in any one session, the more benefit you will get. By doing the tai chi form, you are working on body alignment and *chi* circulation. The number of times you do the form is up to you, but three in a row is a good daily minimum and there is no maximum. Just doing one form is beneficial but this will not bring you maximum benefit nor will it enable you to improve your practice. The first time through the short form is a warm-up and should take about 13 minutes (the first long form should take 30 minutes). Each subsequent execution of the form should be proportionately lower, and the speed should be a minute to a minute-and-a-half slower.

For a beginner, doing the short form once in 15 minutes is a challenge. However, an advanced student would be merely warming up after doing it twice over. When I was on the swim team in high school, we would do 20 laps to warm up. That alone would be plenty of exercise for an average recreational swimmer. The idea of the continuous form is that the first couple of rounds are for warm-up, and the following rounds are for conditioning and advancement. The idea of completing an increasing number of forms as the student becomes more advanced is part of the concept of the continuous form.

### 5.12
### What should our state of mind be while doing the tai chi form? Are we visualizing the *chi* flow?

Contrary to popular belief, the flow of *chi* should never be visualized during tai chi. Doing so will yield fewer benefits from your practice. Remember, *chi* flows through the body, it is not pushed. Doing tai chi improves the body's alignment to facilitate the flow of *chi*. The tai chi movements are movements of self-defense, and to execute them properly you must focus on the meaning of the move. If you are to visualize anything, it would be an opponent. Thus doing the form is a kind of shadowboxing. Through practice you will do the form more correctly and, due to improved alignment, your *chi* will flow better. On the other hand, if you try to do it in reverse, as it were, and ignore the meaning of the move to move, you will actually stifle the *chi*. Your mind will act as a force on *chi* flow, obstructing it.

Instead, learning tai chi involves an awareness of alignment. Are you tucked in? Are you round? Are you balanced? Are you able to go from one move to another with ease? If yes, it means the body alignment is correct and the correct muscles and tendons are being used. If no, the whole frame is not moving correctly. This is why tai chi practitioners must become aware of the whole body connection and not focus on the *chi* circulation.

At a more advanced level, when you know the form and know how to execute it correctly, do it fast. But even when you do the fast form, you don't focus on the flow of *chi*. Instead, the mindset for the fast form should also be like shadowboxing. Are you yielding? Are you attacking? Are you punching? Are you kicking? Are you smooth? You must be very alert and responsive. These are all the things to work on. You never need to worry about *chi* circulation. In fact, it would get in the way. For example, suppose you want to strike with maximum power. Your mind will have the intent for that strike and the *chi* will make it happen. The *chi* will follow your intent — you don't have to visualize it.

### 5.13
### There is more to practicing the fast form than just doing the form faster. What else should we concentrate on?

First, learn to do the form slowly, focusing on relaxation, deep breathing, *tan tien* power, and so on. Execute each move with precision, balance and smoothness, paying close attention to body alignment. At this stage, the goal is to learn the correct structure of tai chi. This is the first step of training.

Next, refine the execution of the moves by learning their application and doing them at a faster speed. In this practice, the aim is to move as fast as possible. Here, the focus is on the meaning of the moves, such as how to strike with power and to yield correctly. It is the same as shadowboxing. Imagine an opponent in front of you while doing the form. At this stage, the goal is to attain power. Once the fundamentals of body alignment are down pat, train for speed.

In slow practice, the mind can be relaxed. It is more internally focused for the purposes of self-cultivation. When moving fast in fighting applications, the mind needs to be alert. It needs to connect the internal to the external instantly, getting the body in correct alignment to deliver power. Only in this way can the form be executed seriously with martial intent. A good fighter enjoys good health and longevity because his nervous system is well exercised. In fact, tai chi slows down the aging process.

### 5.14
### Is it ever a good idea to break up the form to work on specific moves or sections?

You should know the whole form from top to bottom and be able to do the form as one long movement with pauses. However, some parts of the form are more difficult than others to execute, like Single Whip or Fair Lady Works the Shuttle. It is necessary to work on specific moves or sections in order to perfect them. As part of your daily practice, take the time to concentrate on doing one section or move over and over. It is just like a pianist practicing to play a piece of Mozart; he can play the whole piece, but finds one part difficult and drills that section over and over again to get it right. Likewise, you should always aim to improve your form by concentrating on sections. For example, repeat Grasp Bird's Tail for an hour every day for a week and you will improve that portion of the form and, as a result of your effort, your whole form will improve.

### 5.15
### Is the tai chi form continuous from beginning to end without stopping?

The form appears to the casual observer as nonstop motion since some part of the body is always moving. However, to the careful observer, the form is actually a series of waves. Each movement of the form is initiated from the center of the waist, which is called the *tan tien* (the center of the waist, see questions 2.20, 6.5). At the completion of each move, the *tan tien* stops but the hands or feet, depending on the particular move, will continue. Executing the form in this way follows the tai chi principles of alignment discussed throughout this text. If you read the tai chi classics, you see that the tai chi principles are summed up in the old masters' descriptions of the waist as "the pole" or "the axle" of the movement (*TCCP&P,* pp. 57, 82 & 84). Understanding this idea and applying it in practice is difficult.

It is like a whip. To use a whip, the handle is moved and then remains motionless while the end of the whip continues moving. If the body is a whip as it does the form, the *tan tien* is the handle and the fingers (or toes, depending on the move) are the ends of the whip. Each move is initiated from the *tan tien*, the handle of the whip, and finds expression at the end of the whip. When doing the form, the *tan tien* should pause noticeably but some part of the body continues to move — perhaps just the fingers and toes. This whip-like movement is more evident when the form is done fast. Doing tai chi from top to bottom without pausing the *tan tien* is incorrect.

Put another way, the series of movements linked together as the form is just like an essay or musical composition. Essays have sentences and musical scores have phrases. Each movement is a sentence and the whole form is an essay. As in an essay or musical score, there are breaks to separate sentences and phrases. Initiation in the *tan tien* begins the phrase and, for example, strikes are like exclamation points completing the sentence.

### 5.16
### Should the tai chi form be done at the same height?

Yes, the tai chi form should be done at the same height throughout the whole form. In terms of training and improving health using the form, the tai chi form should be done several times a day for a long time, as mentioned above. The first time through the form the body is just warming up. On the second repetition of the form, your stance should be a little lower and a little wider and, again, maintain that height throughout the form. If you have time, do the form a third time and go a little wider, a little lower, a little slower. The idea is that, with each repetition of the form, your body is warmer and more relaxed and you can do the form lower and slower. Now, each person is different. Since lower is more difficult, each person's degree of being lower is going to be different. Make sure you remain relaxed. Don't go lower than you can handle. If you are straining, then you are not receiving benefit from doing the form.

### 5.17
### Will doing the form slowly and correctly over a long period of time give me great internal power and speed?

Yes. The slower the better. As with massage, you want a slow penetrating massage, not a fast rub. Doing the form slowly is like giving the body a slow massage that charges the body's battery while enabling the *chi* to penetrate deeply into the tissues and bones. As in *nei kung*, doing the form slowly makes the body more integrated and stronger. It also integrates the mind and body. I often compare this to a bear; the bear is strong and powerful because its body is connected. Tai chi makes your body like a bear's body. As it says in the classics, "extreme softness can later become extreme hardness" (*TCCP&P,* p. 81). If you practice correctly, with the proper alignment, the body will maintain proper alignment when doing the form fast. The body will have a flow to it as it moves, while internally the *chi* will radiate from the *tan tien* to the whole body. You feel good, full of energy, and powerful. This to me is the beauty of tai chi.

### 5.18
### Why is the *qua* so important?

The two most important motions of the body in executing tai chi originate from the waist and from the *qua*. The waist allows twisting and spiraling in the upper body, while the *qua* governs our lower body connection. The waist controls the hands, and the *qua* the legs. Waist power makes a strong punch. The *qua* permits a strong root and kick.

The *qua* connects leg muscles and tendons to the torso. One needs good connection and flexibility in the *qua* region in order to move effectively. When the *qua* is tight, one's movement is hindered. One cannot deliver a high and powerful kick correctly, nor have tai chi footwork strong enough to allow the body to sink down. Without proper *qua* training, getting correct power is not possible.

### 5.19
### Why are some postures done only on one side? Is this unbalanced?

The body is always in balance, but it is not 100% symmetrical. The heart is not exactly in the center. The bone structure seems symmetrical, but really is not. In my opinion, the structures of some of the attacking moves are good for the right hand and others for the left hand.

Single Whip, for example, is done only on one side. However, it is the same for any weapon form. We hold a weapon like the sword in one hand, making the posture asymmetrical. Western fencing is the same way. One side of the body is always forward. There are punching and kicking moves that can be done on both sides. However, right-handed people will not use the left hand for most actions, and vice versa. It is better to have one sharp knife than two dull ones. If symmetry were a problem, the old masters would have addressed it.

In China, they now practice abbreviated forms with mirrored moves on both the left and right side. I do not think this is necessary. On the one hand, people can do whatever they want for exercise and it may be useful for exercise. But, if you want to do tai chi as a martial art, then you have to do the short form and long form in the traditional way.

### 5.20
### Does it become boring to practice the same form every day for the rest of your life? Isn't there something else to learn?

You eat every day and you sleep every day because those activities are essential for your body. Tai chi recharges your body and becomes just as important as eating and sleeping. Just as you look forward to eating and sleeping, you will begin to look forward to tai chi because it keeps your body healthy, and prevents it from becoming stiff or atrophying. The more deeply you experience tai chi, the more it becomes an intrinsic and challenging part of your life.

Over the centuries, tai chi has been treasured as both the embodiment of a sophisticated philosophy and a martial art. To do tai chi correctly involves the coordination of many factors. Cultivating a mind that is calm, alert, and clear, as well as learning to express that state of mind physically through the tai chi movements, is a process which can be refined endlessly. Furthermore, each time you do the form you experience it anew. You are not in the exact same frame of mind, your body is different, and perhaps the conditions of the room you are in are different. You can also consciously work on emphasizing subtle differences in practicing the form. If you execute a certain kick, for example, you can try to do it faster, or with better root, or from a lower stance. Or you may want to focus on yielding skills one day, striking another day, and relaxation on yet another day.

So, doing the form is never experienced as repetitious. Playing the same instrument everyday, for instance, does not bore a musician because he or she is gaining deeper understanding of the art. If you find tai chi boring, you've missed the point. Getting bored is a sign that you don't understand something essential about tai chi. But in the beginning stages of tai chi practice — before it becomes part of your daily routine — you need an open mind. You need to suspend disbelief. The best way to learn is by doing, by experiencing. Empirical evidence is a most valid and indisputable test of what is good for you. In order for you to undergo the rigors of serious training, you need to begin with an inquisitive mind that can be awakened by the deep philosophical insights of the Tao. Then, when you feel good, and your eyes begin to open to the larger possibilities of tai chi, you will want to do more and more. I believe the most difficult hurdle for the student of tai chi is the first few moves. The Horse Stance, which I show students in the very first Tai Chi Class, is the same position that I work on every day myself. Each move of the form is not something you master and then discard for something more advanced. Just because a principle or movement is simple does not mean it is easy to master. Simple truths are often the most challenging.

### 5.21
### If tai chi is a complete martial art, why should I also practice meditation, *chi kung* and *nei kung*?

To excel in certain areas of tai chi, to get to the maximum power and ability, you need to work on specific details from many branches. The better you learn these extensions and supports for tai chi, the better your tai chi becomes. Though it may be true that you already know tai chi very well, like a physicist gaining deeper knowledge about chemistry, biology and math, you support the core discipline with study of its branches.

Though tai chi contains everything, if you wanted to have more internal power you would choose to do more *nei kung*. *Nei kung* is beneficial for many areas of health. Doing meditation will help you keep a clear mind. If you need to focus on breathing and improving stamina, my *Eternal Spring Chi Kung* will help. Of course, excelling in any or all of these will help your tai chi immensely.

### 5.22
### I've completed the short form and a correction. What should I do next?

At this point, you should try Push-Hands and Fighting I Classes. In Push-Hands Class, you learn how to sense, deflect and redirect your opponent's power; in other words, you learn how "four ounces deflects a thousand pounds" (*TCCP&P,* p. 74). This principle and the skills of push-hands make tai chi different from all other fighting systems. In Fighting I, we work on the tai chi form that you've learned and execute the form correctly for fighting applications, training to maximize the power of attacking whether it's punching, kicking or other forms of striking. Both classes build upon your understanding of the tai chi form. Through these classes, your form will improve.

In addition, there is an empty-handed two-person form taught at my school. The *San Shou* Form is a two-person demonstration form. Through it, novices and non-practitioners can see how the tai chi movements can be applied to a fighting situation. Then there are several weapons forms: Flute, Two-Person Stick, Broadsword, and Double-edged Sword. All of these are advanced forms build on the basic tai chi form.

### 5.23
### How does Push-Hands training strengthen the Tai Chi Form?

Push-Hands is a sensitivity training drill done with a partner. Following a set sequence of four moves, Push, Press, Roll Back, and Ward-Off and Hook, the drill trains attacking and yielding with an opponent. Partners must observe the tai chi principles throughout the drill. The repetition of the sequence, the shifting of weight back and forth, and the application of tai chi principles leads to tai chi form improvement. Through this drill, rooting grows stronger and partners can check their alignment against each other. One will not get the kind of experience push-hands offers from doing only the form. Push-hands is necessary training for improving tai chi.

A student must also practice fighting techniques to understand the power of the tai chi form. Without this understanding, the form has no substance.

Without practicing push-hands and fighting techniques, one cannot really know tai chi, and therefore, practice will remain on a superficial level. Push-hands and fighting techniques are part of advanced training and allow the student to understand the essence of tai chi.

### 5.24
**I've read several books on push-hands and they all discuss it as a competition between two people to see who can maintain their root and balance. Why don't we ever play this game in class? What is the point of push-hands?**

Push-Hands is the intermediate step between learning the form and being able to fight using tai chi. Students at CK Chu Tai Chi are encouraged to take Push-Hands Class after learning the form and before (or while) taking Fighting I (which does not involve partner work). Push-hands is not an end in itself and, by itself, will not prepare you to fight. If you spend a lot of time trying to uproot each other with games, you do gain something — it is fun to compete. However, losing yourself in the game often means losing sight of the goal of push-hands and losing attentiveness to technique. In push-hands games, the person who is stronger and bigger wins, not the person with perfect execution of principles. So, if you play push-hands to see who wins you are wasting time since that is known in advance.

At CK Chu Tai Chi, I prefer spending time on development, on using push-hands to improve the body's ability to follow tai chi principles. Done correctly, push-hands improves bodily alignment (which leads to improvement of your tai chi form practice), and your sensitivity, which is useful later in fighting. If you can stick to a person and follow a person, that is beneficial. This makes it possible to begin to understand the movements of the form and what, for example, the hands are doing at particular junctures.

As you practice push-hands, just as with your tai chi form, you should be able to do it faster and faster without compromising principles. In my opinion, doing push-hands correctly is difficult in itself. When there are competitions, the big guy wins if he just has to root a little bit. Just because he is big and can win at push-hands does not make him a good fighter. Our purpose at CK Chu Tai Chi is to train you to be a fighter. Push-hands is a means to that end, not an end in itself. Otherwise, you can beat people at push-hands but never develop true fighting skills. I think games are acceptable so long as you don't overdo it, which would be a waste of your time. We have to be selective in terms of self-defense and self-cultivation. For example, why don't we spend time on grappling techniques? You should know a little bit about that, but it is more important to develop internal power and take punishment as well as be able to deliver a strong attack and get away from a strong attack. That is the priority. Anything that distracts you from that is a waste of time.

### 5.25
### What are some of the main differences between the way people train today and the way they trained in the past?

In the old days, men needed kung fu to fight on battlefields, both with bare hands and with weapons. Kung fu was a necessary part of their lives. They had to train very seriously to defend against their enemies. Obviously, kung fu is no longer as necessary today as it was in the olden days of hand-to-hand combat. Specifically, training methods in the past emphasized drilling and sparring, with the form reserved only for those at the level of master. Now, it is just the reverse. For us, learning tai chi is to train for health and self-defense; but in reality, there is seldom a need to use it. Therefore, training is never quite as rigorous as it was in ancient times.

However, tai chi is still a sophisticated and high-level martial art. It is a form of art — the art of fighting, of 'deflecting a thousand pounds with four ounces,' on both physical and mental planes. Tai chi also provides a good philosophy of life; it teaches adaptability and going with the flow, or how best to position ourselves and exert minimal force to deal with adversaries. Tai chi is also an art form like painting or music, something that can be done for personal satisfaction.

What sets tai chi apart, however, is that it also has practical benefits for daily life. When the form is done correctly, it promotes well-being. Through practice of the form, coordination and the ability to yield (both mentally and physically) improves. This fosters greater perspective and clarity about life and more energy to do things. Thus, it gives longevity by optimizing the life force. Tai chi practitioners feel healthy, strong, and youthful, and have no need to rely on medications.

For this reason, I consider tai chi to be one of the most valuable treasures of Chinese culture. It is more precious than painting or sculpture. Although beautiful works of art are great, they will not mean anything to a sick person. For a healthy person, on the other hand, tai chi has great practical value. Tai chi also helps a person discover his or her individual Tao, or life essence.

Tai chi is an art form, but with tai chi, the product of the art is one's self. It is not something external to one's body, as in the other arts. The goal of tai chi is better physical and mental health for the artist. Through tai chi a person gains more physical energy and a more optimistic view of the world, which slows the aging process. It is good for the people doing tai chi and good for the people around them. I consider this kind of art to be indispensable for all of us.

This is why I love the art. It is a privilege to learn and appreciate tai chi, and to show its beauty to others. Although it is not needed for the battlefield, I hope everyone will still appreciate the martial value of tai chi as well as its health benefits.

### 5.26
### Some practitioners of hard style kung fu wear weighted hand bands or wrist weights to increase their strength. Should we do this while practicing tai chi?

There is nothing wrong with using weights for certain hand strengthening exercises. As a matter of fact, many people, especially women, probably need more muscle training, but wearing a hand band while practicing tai chi is not a good way to train the muscles. The reason is that, in tai chi, you move the entire body from the *tan tien*. The *tan tien* is like the handle of a whip. Any kind of weight added to your hands affects the whip-like motion of the energy flow, making the wave of energy move differently and not as effectively. There are many different ways to increase your power and strength, but wearing wrist weights during tai chi is not one of them.

### 5.27
### What's the best way to train?

I think it best to be a little bit methodical and set up goals: one day emphasize tai chi, one day *nei kung*, one day meditation, and one day *Eternal Spring*. Another thing is to set realistic goals. For example, do the Horse Stance for five minutes every day, for two weeks. Then after that, increase the duration. The Horse Stance and Playing P'i P'a are the most fundamental exercises for aligning the body. If you are interested in self-defense, fighting techniques or tournaments, you should make a solid schedule for building your endurance and internal power. In the old days there were a lot of tournaments, which made students practice more seriously. You can still train as if you're working towards a tournament. This way you put a carrot in front of yourself. If you are a beginner, you can use the training program from the back of *The Book of Nei Kung*, or set up your own schedule for practicing tai chi or *Eternal Spring*. Once in a while, review your progress and take a serious and realistic look at it. This way you can chart your progress. However, don't be uptight about it. If your body is not ready for the goal your mind has set, you must reassess your goals and listen to your body. Improvement comes gradually. Over time, you will be able to look back and see progress. Suppose you could do only five minutes of Horse Stance and now you can do 25 minutes. That's a big accomplishment.

Why do this? You do it for yourself first, and then so that you can help other people. Also, at my school, there is a test for students at the beginning level or intermediate level for tai chi and *Nei Kung*, and you should look into that and look for the challenge. So far only a few students have taken it but they have gotten great benefit. Students should check in the office to get the program for testing and the guidelines.

### 5.28
### What is the ultimate goal of practicing?

To obtain your own treasure, which is the best 'you' possible. Many masters have thought deeply about tai chi and have determined the principles to be followed in order to receive maximum benefit. It's up to you to love and appreciate tai chi. The practice itself is an infinite challenge, and the body is constantly rewarded with physical and mental benefits along the way. Through tai chi training, a person becomes centered and able to maintain a positive mood; with that comes good health and a long life. During the *Nei Kung* workshop, I always say that after doing *nei kung* we feel very strong and positive. Being able to laugh at every situation in life — that is positive thinking. That is what *nei kung* does to us. When we're healthy and strong, nothing bothers us. We see things differently when we are healthy from when we are not healthy. People around us may be playing games with life, but we don't participate. Although we can laugh, we're very serious about living. Life is too short to be playing games. It is better to live a healthy life.

Tai Chi is not just techniques for self-defense or overcoming your opponent. It's not just a physical exercise. Tai chi is a way of life. In addition to healing, it gives us positive energy for the mind and body. That's the beauty of tai chi, you could say. The treasure is in our body, not outside. An artist spends a lot of time and effort on a painting to make it beautiful. People should spend as much time on their own bodies to make them living works of art.

### 5.29
### How can a person undertake to do tai chi "perfectly"?

Don't think about being perfect all the time. Instead, do tai chi as best you can and enjoy the journey — pursuing the art of movement while cultivating yourself. Otherwise you may become obsessed with perfection and become frustrated. That will actually hinder your progress. It is important to pace yourself. Learning tai chi is a long-term project. If you think of it as something you will do for the rest of your life, you can avoid being overly judgmental about your short-term results. This makes practicing more enjoyable and achieving your goals easier.

### 5.30
### How can we overcome the inertia of not practicing tai chi, when we know tai chi is good for us?

Many who know that tai chi is good for health will practice up to a certain point, but then experience resistance to doing it. This occurs, in part, because the level of improvement that comes from regular practice cannot be readily measured, especially when compared to something like weightlifting where biceps increase by half an inch a month later. Practicing tai chi makes a person feel good but it's hard to track progress. Also, distractions occur and I often hear students say, "Whenever I come to Tai Chi and *Nei Kung* Classes I feel really good. But it seems something always comes up that prevents me from coming." It's easy to find excuses.

### 5.31
### How can we make practice a priority?

I always try to make a point about how we go to work because we're obligated to, yet when it comes to taking care of ourselves we tend to slack off. The truth is that we should keep up our daily practice, and it should be just as important as our job. If we're not healthy and centered we cannot perform well in our job anyway. We should consider our daily practice and coming to classes as a necessity. Just as we have to eat and we have to sleep, so we "have to" practice tai chi. It shouldn't be seen as some kind of an optional activity.

### 5.32
### How does negative thinking keep us from practicing?

Oftentimes, we do some tai chi and realize it's good for us, but don't stick with it for one reason or another. We may have excuses like, "It's not my fault. The teacher isn't paying attention to me. I don't see much progress in a short time." Or you name it. We can find hundreds of excuses. The student should understand that the teacher is really only an advisor. A Taoist teacher is always willing to help. But first we ourselves must value tai chi and the treasure we are seeking in the practice. Otherwise, we'll quickly lose the spirit of seeking and lose sight of the beauty of tai chi, meditation, *chi kung*, and *nei kung*. Then the practice becomes boring and we no longer have total faith in the system. This kind of a negative mindset can easily snowball and drag us in the wrong direction, just as the positive outlook will pull us in the right direction. It's a dangerous situation. We have to pull ourselves out of it.

### 5.33
### How do we cultivate a positive mindset?

Just as the body has to exercise physically, the mind has to have exercise in positive thinking. Meditation will help you do just that. I suggest you take a meditation class and use the *Chu Meditation* book as a guide. And ask a lot of questions. I'll give you a good example of why this is so important. Death rates increase among people who have retired and are not involved in meaningful activities. Why is that? If we do not keep the body and mind stimulated, the mind goes into a negative mode and deteriorates very fast. There's a Chinese saying that this kind of training is like rowing a boat upriver. If you stop, the water will push you back down. We must keep rowing and never stop. Our life is like that: we need continuous mental stimulation.

### 5.34
### If we only have 45 minutes to an hour per day to dedicate to *nei kung*, tai chi and *Eternal Spring*, should we split our time among those practices?

Emphasize one aspect each day. One day you may want to do *nei kung* for 45 minutes and do a few minutes of the rest. The next day you can do more tai chi, then the next day more *Eternal Spring*. All practices are connected with one another, so you can alternate them daily.

For the best results, it is crucial to have a practice routine. At a minimum, your routine should consist of doing the tai chi form for fifteen minutes to half an hour a day, and sitting meditation fifteen minutes to half an hour every day. Weekly, you should do a minimum total of two hours of *Eternal Spring* and two hours of *nei kung* a week.

### 5.35
### What if we have physical pain and don't feel like practicing?

We may complain that our hip or back or some other part of our body hurts. I would say that our body hurts all the time, and that it's supposed to. If we don't use our body it will end up hurting even more. I fell off a horse close to fifteen years ago. It was such a bad fall that my body was paralyzed for a few days. I didn't see a doctor. I healed myself, though not 100%. I still feel it from time to time. And if I don't work on it, I know it's going to get worse. Everybody has something to work on. Professional athletes all have that, too. If we don't use the body, our problems can only get worse. That should give us the drive to say, "I have to work harder." One student who is about 70 years old has a hip problem. Every time she finishes a class she says she feels much better. But when she isn't coming to class she goes back into a negative mode. Now, I can only offer suggestions, but I hope you will read them and reread them as reminders the next time you don't feel like practicing.

### 5.36
### In what order should I practice meditation, *nei kung* and tai chi?

Most beginners should practice in the morning and in the following order: meditation, *Eternal Spring*, *nei kung*, tai chi form and then tai chi application. With this order you warm up your body slowly. That allows you, later on, to go faster and faster.

For beginners, sometimes meditation can be difficult in the morning because there may be some stress from the day before and the mind cannot concentrate. In this situation, it is best to begin with Horse Stance. After several minutes of Horse Stance, walk around to neutralize the body. Then start your practice routine.

### 5.37
### I live far from the city and can only come to tai chi class for corrections occasionally. What is the best way to enhance my practice?

Get the *Chu Tai Chi: Complete Short Form Instruction & Theory* DVD and watch it at least once or twice a week. In a session separate from your daily workout, watch one section of the form, such as from the Commencement to Single Whip, and practice the movements for 15 minutes or more. Do this over the course of a month or so. Then move on to the next section until you've worked through the whole form (see question 5.14).

Occasionally, watch me demonstrate the complete form in the last section of the DVD. It is important that you watch the form demonstration on a regular basis so that you get the feeling and the spirit of tai chi movement. The feeling and spirit are difficult to express in words. By watching the form many times over, your mind will absorb and store the feeling and spirit at a subconscious level.

In fact, I suggest this practice of observation to every student even if he or she takes classes regularly. For most students, "head suspended," "concave chest," "tucked in," "roundness," and "initiate from the *tan tien*" may be possible to execute separately and independently, but students may not be able to unify these separate aspects in smooth, integrated movements. They are not yet able to embody the intricacy or the spirit of tai chi, so to speak. I recommend that all students watch my demonstrations to see how all these elements are integrated in the form. By observing closely, students can compare themselves to the model and see what can be improved.

### 5.38
### After taking two or three classes consecutively in the evening, sleep is difficult. Do you recommend any sort of "cool down" breathing techniques or other exercises to help ease the body into sleep?

After doing tai chi and other exercises, the body is charged up and full of *chi* ready for use. The body is in an active mode instead of a resting mode. This can make it difficult to fall asleep. One easy way to "cool down" the system is to take a long, hot bath. It helps the system change gears from ready to restful, and reassigns the chi to internal healing rather than to activity.

Relax in the tub and empty the mind as in meditation practice. This helps put the body into the sleeping mode. In winter's dry weather, it is also a good idea to use a lotion to keep the skin from drying out after your bath. When you lie down in bed, continue to stay relaxed. There is no need to pressure yourself about how or when you will fall asleep. Sleep will come naturally when the body is ready. Finally, I suggest that you not eat or drink after class, or after your bath.

# VI. TAI CHI, CHI KUNG & NEI KUNG

## 6.1
### What is *chi kung*?

Any exercise that specifically deals with *chi* circulation and is done regularly over a long period of time is *chi kung*. As laid out in chapter 2, *chi* is the "life force." Everyone has it. In fact, a body is alive if it's making and circulating *chi*; it is dead if it's not. The human body is strong and healthy when its *chi* is strong; the body is weak when its *chi* is weak. *Chi* has to be present, and *chi* also has to circulate. If *chi* is missing in the body, say in an organ, the *chi* will not circulate there and the organ will become diseased. A person's health depends on the quantity of *chi* being produced and circulating in the body. Improving the amount and circulation of *chi* in the body is necessary for good health because *chi* is healing energy. If the amount of *chi* can be increased and if it can be circulated, then the weak organ or joint can be renewed. That is the goal of *chi kung*, a system of general exercise isolating single aspects of the generation of *chi*. For example, *chi kung* has exercises in which a person engages in deep breathing and concentrates solely on that. This focus increases *chi* and circulates it. Other exercises focus on improving the alignment of the skeleton, which is also beneficial for *chi* — the better the alignment, the better the circulation of *chi*. My system of *chi kung* is called *Eternal Spring*, a name taken from a line in the tai chi classics; "you are practicing tai chi... for a prolonged life — like an eternal spring" (*TCCP&P*, p. 91). *Eternal Spring Chi Kung* has elements of *nei kung* in its program.

## 6.2
### What is *nei kung*?

Literally, *nei kung* means "internal work." Doing *nei kung* means you are working on the body down to the cellular level. This training makes all the body's cells, tendons, bones, and fascia very strong, from the inside out. When this happens, the body can be so strong that it is as if a "muscle shield" is protecting it: as if you are wearing an elastic suit that covers the whole body. High level *nei kung* is called the "Iron Vest" or "Golden Bell" system because this shield surrounding the body becomes so strong it is nearly impenetrable and thus able to withstand a great deal of punishment. In addition, *nei kung* trains your mind to be relaxed, flexible, and very responsive. This training harmonizes the subconscious mind and body. You are very relaxed, very strong, and the whole body is integrated as one unit from low to high level. This depends on the dedication of the individual. *Nei kung* has been passed down from ancient times and, to me, it is a true treasure of the martial art system.

### 6.3
### Please explain the difference between *chi kung* and *nei kung*.

Both types of exercises increase and circulate *chi*. *Chi kung* exercises occur while standing in one place to facilitate healing through a focus on breathing and stretching in a certain way, but the postures are not held long. *Nei kung* is like '*chi kung* plus' because while working on the *chi*, mind power and mind relaxation enable *chi* to penetrate the internal organs, the bones, the tendons, the muscles, and the nervous and circulatory systems. In *nei kung* certain postures are held for a long time. The result of practicing *nei kung* over a long span of time is a body so strong and flexible it is impenetrable to attack. This is useful for the martial artist, since he doesn't get hurt when hit. *Chi kung* does not have this effect. For more information on my systems of *chi kung* and *nei kung*, see *Eternal Spring Chi Kung* and *The Book of Nei Kung (Nei Kung)*.

### 6.4
### If *nei kung* is a more intense level of developing *chi*, why bother with *chi kung* at all?

At my school, students work on four basic subjects: meditation, tai chi form, *chi kung*, and *nei kung*. Fighting and weapons training come on top of these basics. As in any school, you take different courses to focus on specific topics. If you take a geology, chemistry, or astronomy course, maybe later you will use the information you learn in them to specialize in physics. You need to know all related fields and a broad knowledge of things to be good at one field. All of the subjects taught at my school are interrelated and all work together for the purpose of making a healthy, whole body. To improve your health by increasing your *chi* you need to do both *chi kung* and *nei kung*. For most people, it is best to focus on *chi kung* at first until they are ready for *nei kung*. When they are ready to practice *nei kung*, they should not stop doing *chi kung*.

My *chi kung* system (called *Eternal Spring*) and my *Nei Kung* system complement each other. In fact, *Eternal Spring* is designed to lead to *Nei Kung*; when practicing at home, students can start the *Nei Kung* series when they get to the Horse Stance in the *Eternal Spring* series (doing Pivoting Into Bow Stances later). *Eternal Spring* should be part of your training program because in that series you can focus on things that you cannot focus on during *Nei Kung*. For example, development of correct deep breathing is essential to tai chi, but due to the complexity of the *Nei Kung* exercises, it is difficult to focus just on breathing. Many students readily understand the importance of breathing, but they don't work on it. *Eternal Spring* gives you the opportunity to work just on diaphragm breathing. *Eternal Spring* also works on alignment, loosening up the joints, relaxation, and mind-body connection. *Nei Kung* is a little more advanced because you need to have more correct alignment to do the stances, and then you need the physical and mental stamina to hold the stances for a long time. Breathing is not unimportant; it just isn't a focus in *Nei Kung*. Rather, the focus is on holding the stances in order to put the skeleton into better alignment. Stance training, as is done in *nei kung*, is good for *chi* circulation, balance, and improving the tai chi form.

I devised *Nei Kung* first and then developed *Eternal Spring*, in part, to focus on those areas of development not in the *Nei Kung* regimen. The two systems complement each other and people should do both in order to have the chance to focus on what each exercise is designed for. Let's suppose you just do *Nei Kung*: then your diaphragm breathing will not be as strong and your joints not as loose. Tai chi training is a package of meditation, *chi kung*, *nei kung*, and the form. Some parts of *Eternal Spring* may be basic, but that does not mean they are not important. The elements of the package are interrelated, becoming integrated in the tai chi form, in fighting, and in daily life.

### 6.5
### Can the development of *chi* be felt during *nei kung* and *chi kung*?

Just when and how intensely *chi* is felt during exercise differs from person to person. In general, you should feel heat in the *tan tien* first (see 2.20). This is usually the first place students feel heat as they do the first few *Eternal Spring Chi Kung* exercises or during Roaring Lion. You should also notice heat there as you become comfortable with the basic 20-minute Horse Stance of *Nei Kung*. As training in Horse Stance progresses, the next area many students feel heat is in the lower back. Eventually, after the sensation of heat in these and other areas becomes a normal part of your training, you will feel heat travel between the lower and middle tan tiens along the meridian that links the two regions. This will occur without any direction on your part. To repeat what I've said elsewhere, do not try to speed up this process by visualizing the movement or anything like that — just let it happen when it happens.

### 6.6
### Other teachers say the toes should be turned out during *chi kung* exercises generally but also during Horse Stance specifically, but you say 'toes in.' Why is this?

In any art, excellence can be attributed to certain details without which the work would be less successful — like a secret ingredient or special technique used in preparing a recipe. Many Chinese restaurants feature "Monk's dish" on their menus, for example, but it will taste so-so when prepared by one cook, and exceptionally delicious when prepared by another.

In Cantonese, these secret details are called *"bay kuk."* In the martial arts, *bay kuks* were treasured knowledge revealed to only a select few. You can say all the principles of *nei kung* were considered secret at one time. "Toes in" is one such *bay kuk*.

Turning the toes in is a detail of aligning the body to facilitate the flow of *chi* that not many know about. If you study the photographs in *"chi kung"* and *"nei kung"* books, you will see many instructors posing with arched back, toes turned out, and knees turned in. Eventually, they, and their students, hurt themselves and the first thing injured is the knee. Some of these teachers have invented new exercises to correct the knee problems they created for themselves by unknowingly doing the exercises with incorrect alignment. However, if they practiced correctly in the first place, by moving the knee the way it is best moved, they would not need to do this extra work.

Many people have alignment problems in the leg. This is made evident when they bend their knees to do Horse Stance. Their back arches, their knees inevitably go inward (cave in), their toes point out, and their feet will not be flat on the floor. This poor alignment indicates poor *chi* circulation and is accompanied by shallow breathing. Fixing this alignment with tai chi training is a matter of consistently aligning the body correctly while practicing and then eventually the alignment will become natural to the body. First, during *nei kung* or *chi kung* exercise, make sure the toes are pointed in. By this I do not mean you should stand pigeon-toed. Rather, turning your toes in *slightly* is good for your *chi* circulation and for improving your alignment. Over time, you may turn your toes in less and less. But the process depends on the state of your alignment and on the shape of the foot. After all, each person has a different bone structure so each person's angle for the toe will be different. Another benefit from turning the toes in is that this helps to put the weight on the outer edges of the foot. This strengthens the arch of the foot.

The aim, here, is to explain how "toes in" help a person improve his or her alignment during training. But I want to be clear: the ideal is a relaxed foot that is flat on the floor with the toes pointing straight ahead and the knees directly over the toes as in the diagram in *The Book of Nei Kung* (p. 23), especially while you are doing the tai chi form. If your foot is not flat, you will not be able to balance too well and then you will not be able to do the tai chi form well, let alone fight. As I remind my students, the rule to apply is relaxation. If you are not relaxed in the Horse Stance, something is out of place somewhere — check your feet.

### 6.7
### Is it important to follow the order of the exercises in *Eternal Spring* and *Nei Kung* books?

Yes, follow the sequence laid out in *The Book of Nei Kung* but feel free to stop at any point. The sequence of these exercises is designed to repair and rejuvenate the body. One can be a little more flexible with the *Eternal Spring* series. For example, along with the 12 foundational exercises, there are supplemental exercises — these can be added in or not, depending on how a person feels. Also, *Eternal Spring* exercises can be used to warm up the body before doing *Nei Kung*, tai chi, or Fighting Class. With experience and knowledge of your body, you will discover which specific exercises you should do given the time you have to prepare and the activity you wish to be ready for. But *Nei Kung* is a recipe for health, and the exercises work together to achieve the desired aim of good health, so just follow the directions.

### 6.8
### What is the concept behind the order of the *Eternal Spring* series?

There are 12 exercises in the *Eternal Spring Chi Kung* series. These exercises break down into three sections of four exercises each. They are:
    Dragon Claws, Fish Leaps Up, Yawning Lion, Sleeping Lion
    Roaring Lion, Frog Stance, Golden Rooster, Crane Stretches Wings
    Shifting Frog, Easy Horse Stance, Tai Chi Opening, Pivot into Bow Stance.

When you are first learning *Eternal Spring*, concentrate on the first section. While all the exercises develop flexibility, alignment, and breathing, the first section focuses on the practice of diaphragm breathing and opens the body up. In this section, the beginner explores correct diaphragm breathing and the most advanced student furthers his or her mastery of diaphragm breathing. The second section contains advanced techniques for further development of correct diaphragm breathing, like the rapid fire of Roaring Lion, as well as some stance training. In time, the postures of the second set lead to the body breathing from the diaphragm involuntarily. The last section charges up the body, preparing it for doing the tai chi form.

    *Eternal Spring* is a recipe for health and, if followed, it will yield results. The sequence and timing are both important. When you practice, don't rush through the exercises. Rather, do each one as correctly as possible for as long as you need to. If you have a limited amount of practice time, you should concentrate on doing one section only (preferably the first) rather than rushing through the whole series. *Eternal Spring* teaches the fundamentals of tai chi while helping you to improve your alignment.

### 6.9
### What is the concept behind the order of the *Nei Kung* series?

Think of the body as a beautiful castle on a hill that needs reconstruction and remodeling. The process of exploring and repairing the castle will take time and necessarily depends on a step-by-step approach. First, the front gate and main wall must be very strong since the integrity of the whole castle depends on the strength of the main fortification. The Horse Stance is the first exercise in *Nei Kung* because it strengthens the whole body (or, to switch metaphors, it is like the motor in a car — you want the motor fine-tuned). Doing Horse Stance, the body warms up; the body's battery is recharged; and the lower back is improved, as is your general alignment. Having warmed up and opened the body, it is then possible to proceed to the details of proper alignment. But it is not a one-time fix. You have to do the Horse Stance consistently in order to rebuild your front gate and main wall.

For communication (that is, *chi* flow) through the castle, there is a main thoroughfare connecting courtyards and buildings. The second exercise in *Nei Kung*, Riding the Wild Horse, improves this circulation system by spreading the *chi* around while relaxing and stretching the muscles. Again, the more you do the exercises, the more your castle will improve. The third exercise moves back to the fortifications (the body's overall integrity) to work on the two side gates with P'i P'a. With Horse Stance, work is being done on the major meridian lines, the big orbit. P'i P'a comes at the body from a different direction to work the left and right side meridians. As with Horse Stance, after you complete P'i P'a, you once again spread the *chi* and stretch with exercise number four, the Compass. The Compass involves greater integration of the body as one piece, moving as one unit, but its goals are similar to that of Riding the Wild Horse. Think of it as reconstructing the interior halls and courtyards.

Next, attention is turned to various rooms and decorations. Double Dragons Leap from the Sea, the next exercise in *Nei Kung*, fixes your alignment and also moves *chi* from *tan tien* to the floor and back up to hands. This is a very difficult exercise to do correctly until the body's alignment is fixed. It works on the development of internal striking power by fostering the accelerated movement of *chi* from the *tan tien* to the rear foot on the floor and back out through the hands, resulting in an indestructible power dynamic. The next exercise, Rhinoceros Gazes at the Moon, is rotating the spine to improve flexibility as well as fine-tuning the mechanisms of the body while stimulating the central organs. Work on the castle now moves to the towers; Phoenix Spreads Wings spreads the *chi* from the *tan tien* to the fingertips. In this exercise, the body is flapping its wings — trying to fly. From the towers, we go down to the dungeons, as it were. Hitting the Tiger exercises the *qua*. Finally, the regimen ends in the throne room with Owl Turns Head as a final adjustment to the whole body focusing on the head-body connection.

*Nei kung* develops internal power, not just stronger muscles. Internal power comes from the whole body being healthy and strong, which is accomplished by doing these exercises. The exercises promote healing, repairing, and strengthening of your muscles, tendons, bones, organs, and cells. By design, the exercises circulate *chi*, strengthen muscles, and align the body in a particular sequence to realize this goal. It is not obvious, but certain movements affect the organs — massaging and healing them — even though they seem to be muscle movements. While all the exercises affect the organs, certain exercises focus on particular organs. For example, the Horse Stance works on the whole body but especially the kidneys, while Phoenix Spreads Wings works on the lungs and heart. So besides charging the body with *chi*, the muscles, tendons and bones are linked together correctly and the whole system is strengthened every time you do the regimen. That is *nei kung*, internal power. By doing *nei kung*, your tendons become more flexible and stronger, your bones denser, stronger and more lively, your muscles more evenly distributed and better able to help the tendons connect the body together, but not with bulging muscles as in weight lifting. Additionally, the organs are nourished and massaged so they can work optimally. Do the series every day and the body will get stronger and stronger with more vitality, reversing the aging process. That is the recipe for health — that is *nei kung*, internal power.

## 6.10
## In between *Eternal Spring Chi Kung* exercises we open our mouths and breathe out audibly. Why do we do this?

During *Eternal Spring* exercises we breathe in and out through the nose and follow the principles of long, deep, small and smooth breathing. It's the same in *Nei Kung*. However, in between *Eternal Spring* exercises we don't do slow breathing. As a matter of fact, we try to breathe out as quickly as possible, so in this case the mouth is open. Sometimes with an open mouth we purposefully make a sound, a "haaaaaa"-type sound with the throat, to work on the respiratory system.

The goal is to train the respiratory system for both slow and fast breathing. It is the same principle as working the cardiovascular system, where we focus on pushing ourselves on both sides of the spectrum, moving from very slow to very fast. The same is true of breathing: go from very slow to very fast. The audible sound is part of the technique used to make the breath come out fast.

Sometimes when a horse breathes out it also makes a sound — a loud "neighing" sound. I think this is the same kind of fast breathing designed to push out as much air as possible.

Many aspects of martial arts were learned by copying animals, and this may be where this breathing technique originated.

## 6.11
## What is the purpose of Roaring Lion in *Eternal Spring*?

Roaring Lion is one of the exercises in *Eternal Spring* that works on fast breathing both in and out. To make the sound "hing" you must close the throat and push some air down quickly to the *tan tien* with the diaphragm moving downward. To make the sound "har" you hit the body at the *tan tien* with the fingers and squeeze the air out through the throat.

Think of it as blowing up a balloon — you want to close the valve so the air will stay in the balloon. Inevitably, some air will come out when you close the valve. It is the same when we make the sound "hing." Some air will go to the lungs with the diaphragm moving downward, and some air will come out through the throat to make the sound "hing." When we make the "har" sound it's like hitting the balloon — the valve will open up and some of the air will come out through the throat.

This "hing-har" exercise works your breathing apparatus in fast mode. It is an exercise for transforming the breathing of air (oxygen) into *chi* — the energy that flows in our system. Even a beginner will feel the body heat up during this exercise. This indicates the body's strong flow of *chi*.

## 6.12
## When we start the Horse Stance, at what height should we be? Should we start low, medium, or high? Why?

The idea is similar to doing the form. Start high with the feet at shoulder width and the knees slightly bent. After several minutes, when the body has warmed up, then it is ready to go lower. An advanced student can go lower every few minutes, repositioning the feet slightly wider apart. The key here is to remain relaxed. When the alignment is correct, the body can be very, very relaxed; it feels as if it can "last forever" in the position. The most important thing is to tuck in the pelvis and bring the knees forward.

A beginner has a tendency to let the knees move away from above the toes toward the back. This is incorrect. The knees should go as far forward as they can with the body's weight in the heels and the heels not lifting off the floor. This is a well-balanced position. Here, the tendons and muscles are being stretched and the center of gravity is in the right place. The body's weight is correctly supported, which allows the *chi* to be strong.

The student should not do a low Horse Stance right away. Listen to your body and make sure it is warmed up first.

### 6.13
### Please explain in more detail the three stages of developing the back in Embracing Horse.

It is advisable for a beginning student to lean forward a lot. Leaning forward is fine as long as the principles laid out in the *Nei Kung* manual, such as the concave chest and tucking in, are followed. In the beginning, the necessary muscles are not yet developed and a person cannot make the back straight correctly. Therefore, early in one's practice, the focus should be on strengthening the lower back by leaning forward, tucking in, and never arching the back.

Once the lower back is stronger and the "tuck" is correct, lean forward less. At this stage, the back should be held in a more upright, straighter position. Now the focus is on the middle back.

Finally, the back is strong enough to hold an even more upright position with a much straighter back. The straighter the back, the better. The spine should be straight with a natural curve, as if it is a string of beads hanging from the ceiling. The same principles should be adhered to: tucking in, knees over the toes, and stress falling on the thighs — not on the knees. As this is a difficult posture to hold, the importance of a correct "tuck" needs to be emphasized.

Different people have different problems, and some problems take longer to be corrected than others. However, the instructions here are a general guide as to how one can strengthen the back, from the bottom up.

### 6.14
### What should "lasting forever" feel like?

Each of us has individual physical and mental limitations. If any part of the body hurts while doing the Horse Stance, it means the body is fixing some type of injury or blockage. If there is pain, hold the position for as long as possible, up to the point it starts to be too painful. Each time you practice you will notice you can hold the position a little longer than the last time. It indicates the body is in the process of healing. Horse Stance is a healing exercise. It puts the body in correct alignment, stretching it in the right places and strengthening the tendons and muscles in the right way, ultimately correcting the body's functioning overall.

### 6.15
### If you are in correct alignment, should your legs be feeling relaxed or is it normal to experience some degree of muscle strain?

It depends on the individual. If one has a totally healthy body, one will feel the strain in the thighs. However, with many people the knees tend to cave in and the stress is felt on the outside of the legs (see question 2.7). For instance, when a woman wears high heels, her body's weight falls on the wrong part of her foot when she walks. When she does the Horse Stance and puts the body in correct alignment, the strain will be felt in the ankles. This is a good sign: it means the ankles are being fixed. Another person may have a lower back problem, perhaps a distortion of the spine from sitting in one position all the time. Horse Stance releases the stress from the back by letting it fall into correct alignment. Suspending the head elongates the spine. It becomes like a suspended string of beads, with each vertebra sitting on top of another without strain.

### 6.16
### During Horse Stance, should I be "doing" anything?

Horse Stance is also a standing meditation. As in sitting meditation, the goal of which is to sit quietly and nothing more, the goal of Horse Stance is to stand quietly. To master the art of standing quietly, there are steps you should keep going through, until you no longer need them and you can just do the Horse Stance. First of all, spot-check yourself by asking a series of questions: Am I suspended enough, loose enough, relaxed enough, tucked in enough, round enough; are my toes pointing in slightly; is the weight of my body on the outside of my feet; are my knees over my toes?

Spot-check your alignment first and then work on deep breathing. Breathe down into the diaphragm and as you inhale, stretch your fingers. When you exhale, relax. Breathe in that manner a few times and then go through your spot-check list again. For example, if your hip is troubling you, try to feel whether it has tightened up, thus turning the toe out and causing misalignment. Bring yourself back in alignment with your checklist. Go back and forth between alignment and focused deep breathing.

Once your alignment has begun to improve and you've become habituated to Horse Stance, or, on the other hand, your mind is working against you too much to do the above, apply sitting meditation techniques: head suspended and breathing down to the *tan tien*, put the mind in the *tan tien*, count to 10, and empty the mind (see *Chu Meditation* for details).

### 6.17
### How can *nei kung* help develop muscle strength in the upper body? Can it substitute for weight training?

*Nei kung* helps build muscle strength in the upper body. However, the exercise doesn't isolate any one specific group of muscles and work on it independently. The primary objective of *nei kung* is to integrate all the body's parts and systems into a single functional unit. The center of the unit is the *tan tien*, from which the power radiates out to every part of the body. *Nei kung* develops the body's overall strength and generative power or ging; weight training develops localized muscle strength or *li*, which is part of ging (see *TCCP&P,* pp. 128-130).

There is nothing wrong with light weight-training. For example, most women have weak upper body muscles and need to develop more *li*. Light weight-training and some push-ups and pull-ups are good exercise for them. However, for any tai chi practitioner, it's important not to overemphasize bodybuilding with weights. This is because it concentrates on just part of the body whereas the goal of tai chi is to strengthen the body as a whole.

There are certain groups of muscles for pulling motions and others for punching motions. Overly developed "pulling" muscles make one muscle-bound, which hinders freedom of movement in combat. The weight of the extra mass slows the speed of motion, and the lack of the *tan tien* connection reduces the power of delivery. It is the coordination of the tendons, not the muscles, that gives speed and power to an attack. The muscles merely support the tendons.

Take an Olympic swimmer, for instance. He needs to have strength, agility and endurance in order to be a competent swimmer. He cannot have bulky muscles that slow down his movement and diminish his coordination. He needs to be able to use the whole body as one unit, just as in tai chi.

Western-style weight training focuses on muscle toning alone. In tai chi, if a student wishes specifically to train the upper body, there are other means to do so without compromising the integrity of the body. He can train his upper body by practicing fighting applications such as punching and sticking. He can also practice weapons like the Broadsword, which has movements that strengthen the tendons and bones of the upper body. Advanced forms of meditation also strengthen the muscles in the upper body.

### 6.18
### Does high-level *chi kung* and *nei kung* training strengthen the body's weakest points like the eyes, kidneys and groin?

The answer is yes. In general, *chi kung* and *nei kung* train the whole body. It is not specifically for the eyes, kidney or groin, but increasing the strength of these parts of the body is one positive side effect of the tai chi exercise system.

*Nei kung* spreads *chi* from the *tan tien* to the rest of the body. This is the natural process. By practicing every day, the body becomes healthier and stronger a little bit at a time. Increased strength will not be too obvious. However, if you check after a *Nei Kung* Class, your eyesight is actually sharper. If you look at a watch before and after, you'll notice that you can see it better afterwards. Your energy makes your eyes stronger in a very short time. There are many, many other examples. Just the other day an 86-year-old student called me and said his hearing had improved. Another student in her late sixties told me her bone density had increased. Her doctor was surprised — usually, your bone density decreases as you get older. Many clear, quantifiable improvements result from *nei kung*, but the improvements are so slow that you may not notice them right away.

### 6.19
### What does one need to watch out for if one is practicing too much *nei kung*?

Too much of anything is not good for the body. When training, be sure to allow for proper rest and recuperation time as well as adequate sleep. Too much too soon will have a reverse effect on the body. Pay attention to how your body feels in order to know how much is enough. Each person is different. If a person's comfort zone for practicing Horse Stance is 20 minutes, he or she should not continue for 2 hours. That would be too much. With internal training like *nei kung*, improvement must be gradual and natural.

### 6.20
### How do *chi kung, nei kung*, and tai chi exercise the organs?

The organs — such as the lungs, the heart, and the kidneys — are never static. They are alive and constantly working, especially during exercise. The movements in *chi kung, nei kung*, and tai chi compress and expand the organs in certain ways, thereby increasing the *chi* circulation and implementing healing of the body.

Certain body alignments, held in a static posture, also benefit the organs. A good example is Horse Stance. It may look like nothing is happening. However, holding the posture stimulates the kidneys and helps to circulate the *chi*. Deep breathing is always good for the lungs. The movement of the diaphragm massages the organs too. It also stimulates the meridians just as acupuncture would. When *chi kung, nei kung*, or tai chi is done correctly, the effects are longer lasting than acupuncture. Using needles, the acupuncturist adjusts the flow of *chi* by stimulating the gates in the meridian system to improve the flow of existing *chi*. In contrast, *chi kung, nei kung*, and tai chi strengthen the muscles and tendons to adjust the alignment of the skeleton so as to generate *chi* and enhance its circulation (see question 2.3).

### 6.21
### Is *nei kung* some kind of bulletproof vest?

Not bulletproof, of course, but amazingly strong. Take the example of one student who had abdominal surgery. The doctor had trouble cutting through the student's stomach with his scalpel. This surprised the doctor because the patient did not have the typical body-builder six-pack muscles, but rather stomach muscles that were evenly distributed and connected: a uniform muscle shield. This student's abdomen was like a tire that was completely even and strong. Like most animals, his muscles were without bulge, but acted as an overall united, connected tissue — with strength like that of the bear. If you visualize a bear, which can look fat, you should also know that it is very flexible, powerful, physically connected, and practically invincible. You will see roundness, connectedness and unified movement in its body. *Nei kung* gives you the body of a bear.

### 6.22
### What is the chief benefit or pay-off for doing *nei kung*?

You will know if *nei kung* is paying off by the results. You will feel good, energized and strong. *Nei kung* fixes the body's alignment, which allows the healing energy of *chi* to flow better. Doing *nei kung* will heal back pain, neck pain, migraine headaches and many other ailments.

There are other benefits of improving *chi* with *nei kung*. You'll think more clearly and have more energy in everyday life. Even your hearing and eyesight will improve (and while it won't heal nearsightedness or farsightedness, you will see more clearly). Another benefit is that the *chi* energy is also sexual energy. Doing *nei kung* makes you feel youthful.

In terms of fighting, you will gain internal power so that when you get punched or struck by an opponent you may hardly feel it. In other words, *nei kung* just strengthens you overall. That is why the art was kept a secret for so long — in order to prevent its use against you. I struggled with this issue myself. In the 1970s, I did not want to openly teach *nei kung* because I wanted my students to have the edge in tournaments. But I changed my mind when I realized that *nei kung* exercises are not only a recipe for health but for longevity, strength and youthfulness that can benefit people in general. To me, it is one of the treasures of ancient Chinese culture.

### 6.23
### Does *nei kung* strengthen the knees?

Absolutely. The moment you begin to hold Horse Stance you are strengthening your joints and kidney area. Most knee problems originate from poor alignment. People with tight hips bend their knees incorrectly. Their knees go inward and twist. A knee cannot bear this kind of strain. A knee is like a finger. It is intended to bend only one way.

Knee injuries are common in the world of sports because the knee is like a shock absorber for the body. Knees can be worn down by running and jumping. Fortunately, *Nei Kung* and *Eternal Spring* make the knees strong and protect them from future abuse.

People often forget that strong knees are also important for a healthy sex life. Good sex, never mind great sex, is a vigorous exercise. Weak knees only hinder that experience. I remember reading about a lone giraffe in the London Zoo. The zookeepers brought in a mate, but the poor giraffe hadn't had sex in some time. After the act, the giraffe couldn't stand up! Its knees were too weak and the animal had to be lifted out with a crane. This story certainly underlines the importance of knee strength.

## 6.24
## What additional *nei kung* exercises are there?

You should have at least five years of regular training before you learn other techniques. If you have been training for a long time, you can try doing Horse Stance lower and lower. Again, this is only something you should try if you have years of experience.

If you don't have a teacher, follow my book. If you shoot an arrow and are even just a little bit off in your aim, your arrow will be way off the mark.

## 6.26
## Are there psychological benefits of doing *nei kung*?

Obviously, tai chi, *chi kung*, and *nei kung* are physical exercises, but humans are not just physical beings. Humans are also made up of emotional and mental dimensions. Each exercise regimen helps fix the alignment of the body, which, as has been said throughout this book, facilitate the *chi* flow, and this has mental and emotional repercussions.

First, doing tai chi requires a level of maturity and self-discipline. It must be done daily and done correctly. Dedication to tai chi makes the mind stronger while improving concentration. Such benefits spill over into other areas of life. Doing tai chi in the morning sets a positive, relaxing tone for the day.

In *nei kung*, particular postures are held for certain amounts of time, which generates *chi* and circulates it to where it is needed the most. Sometimes physical and emotional problems are connected because emotional trauma is registered, a.k.a. remembered, in the body. Thus, the circulation of *chi* to a specific painful area to smooth out that part of the body and physically heal it may also be smoothing out the emotions and the mind. When that happens, pent up emotions are released; this can cause uncomfortable mental pain, as those emotions are released while doing the postures. For healing to occur, you have to go through some pain, physical and mental. The reward is that you are becoming physically, emotionally, and mentally closer to being the ideal you.

The ideal body has no pent-up stress, mentally or physically. But nobody is ideal — everybody has some degree of stress-induced discomfort. Everybody is born with different strengths, weaknesses, and personality attributes, and then each person experiences life differently, accumulating different discomforts with different healing needs. Since each person is unique, each person's *nei kung* experience will be different. But everyone who does *nei kung* will go through a beneficial healing process. The beginner may experience the healing process as discomfort and fatigue in the initial stages. This is part of the process, and you just need to rest and recover. During the second stage, the body will heat up and sweat. Some people will experience emotional healing with further practice and time. Over 40 years of teaching, I've seen all kinds of involuntary releases like shaking, crying, jumping, moaning, and even laughing. Mostly people feel shaking and heat. A small minority of people have extreme reactions, which can be disturbing to others in a classroom situation so it is best that they work this out at home without an audience.

# VII.
# TAI CHI AND MEDITATION

### 7.1
### There are so many different kinds of meditation systems, each with its own philosophy. How do they compare with what you teach?

Meditation has different meanings and purposes for different cultures. In fact, the only thing all forms of meditation have in common is that they are done while one is sitting still.

I practice and teach Taoist meditation. In Taoist meditation, the goal is to sit still for a long time, empty the mind, and relax. This is done while sitting in the lotus position, which creates correct alignment and energy flows, charging up the body. For those who cannot do the lotus position, consult *Chu Meditation* for alternate positions while you undertake a stretching program. It may take you a few years to be able to do the full lotus but that is OK, there is no rush. Those alternate positions will still allow you to gain benefits from sitting meditation. The lotus position is the most efficient position, so you should aim for that by stretching a little bit every day. The main thing is that you improve yourself a little at a time. Taoist meditation refreshes the body and is actually better for the body than going to sleep. You can find step-by-step instructions for Taoist meditation in my book.

### 7.2
### What is Taoist meditation?

It is a physical and mental exercise to make a healthier brain. Taoist meditation is quiet sitting in which you align the body in a certain way, holding that alignment for as long as possible, and breathing from the diaphragm. Through this exercise you will discover who you really are or, in Taoist terminology, discover your path (your individual Tao).

## 7.3
## Is it easy to discover your individual Tao?

Taoist meditation is guided by Taoist philosophy. In class, I teach the Taoist concepts so you will see things from a Taoist perspective. Taoists are flexible, not rigid. A high-level Taoist has a childlike interest in life, is curious, and desires to explore and question things. A Taoist is happy and energetic.

Tao means "the way" or "path." You discover your own way, your own Tao, through a regular and prolonged meditation regimen. Through meditation, your body and mind are more relaxed and calm. As a result, you will be able to discover your own uniqueness, your own Tao.

It can be a challenge to become a Taoist and discover your own Tao, but, as in tai chi, the Taoist way is to strive for the goal without too much struggle. Discovering your Tao through meditation practice should not be looked on as a struggle. Meditation is enjoyable. It is fulfilling. It feels good. Afterwards, it allows you to think freely.

The Taoist tries to be free from the rules made by society, religion and family culture that suppress your Tao. Different cultures pose different challenges to people. Patriarchal cultures, for example, are harder on women and, therefore, women have a more difficult time discovering their Tao, let alone following it. Taoists try to see the essence of life. Too many man-made laws hinder people's progress.

Of course, society's rule-makers and politicians do not encourage this kind of thinking.

They don't see that what's good for one person might not be good for all people. Taoists see things with more clarity and don't waste time playing the games many people play. As Taoists, we prefer to be ourselves and have fun.

## 7.4
## Is meditation an important part of tai chi training?

Meditation is indispensable. It is one of the pillars of tai chi training. Without it, it is impossible to become a high-level practitioner of tai chi.

If you cannot sit still and meditate, you have problems. Your body is not calm. Your mind is racing and not relaxed. You are not "yourself."

Meditation leads to enlightenment. At a high level of practice it is possible to meditate for a long time and reach a new stage of consciousness. At that stage, it will seem as if all secrets are revealed, and everything suddenly seems obvious and clear.

As I wrote in my book, *Chu Meditation*, Taoists have a special name to describe the kind of "true feeling" that comes with the practice of high-level meditation: *Jung Yun* (*Jung* meaning "Real," *Yun* meaning "Person"). The Real Person sees things as they are. You are true to yourself and true to your beliefs. In other words, the *Jung Yun* sees the essence of life and acts accordingly (see *Chu Meditation* pp. 8-9).

Meditation, more than any other practice I've experienced, has revealed to me the essence of life, which is pursuing your own Tao, preserving your health, fulfilling your potential and seeking intrinsic happiness. These benefits have positive effects on everything we do, including tai chi.

## 7.5
## What does meditation have to do with self-defense?

Many aspects of tai chi training are not too obvious to the casual observer. A person might look at someone sitting and meditating and "doing nothing" and ask, "Why are you doing this?" During meditation, a person is seen merely sitting; while in actuality, his or her energy is moving strongly inside the body. When the outside of the body is more static, the inside of the body is more dynamic.

Meditation training has many benefits. It charges the body with healing energy and increases the sensitivity of the body and the mind. You become more centered, calm, sensitive, alert, controlled, and in tune with the situation. Self-defense will come more easily and naturally with no struggle or obstruction to a person who meditates because of the increased health and calmness of mind. This is what the tai chi classics mean when they say high-level goals can be obtained without kung-fu — without working hard and without struggle.

## 7.6
## What's the difference between the standing meditation of Horse Stance and the lotus position of sitting meditation?

Horse Stance, an important posture in *nei kung*, works on alignment. It strengthens the thigh, the hip, the back and increases body connection.

Sitting meditation is also good for alignment, but it lacks the muscle and tendon development of *nei kung*. If you just do sitting meditation, the body won't have the internal power to withstand strong impact from fighting.

The purpose of sitting meditation is to experience clarity of mind as well as development of *chi*. It is less strenuous than Horse Stance and, because of that, it is possible to sit for hours and hours (whereas you cannot do Horse Stance for that long). A long period of sitting meditation is important for the development of *chi*.

## 7.7
## Why is "quiet sitting" good for us?

As society becomes increasingly complex, people feel increasingly pressured. Meditation helps people to function more efficiently by increasing mental clarity. It allows a person to see better where he or she is going in life and discover his or her own nature or Tao. When the mind is preoccupied, the *chi* is blocked from going to the places in the body where it is needed. The goal of Taoist meditation is to put the mind into a neutral state so that the *chi* can flow naturally and heal the body.

## 7.8
## How does having a strong mind help us in our daily life?

When things are good, anyone can feel good. When things are tough, meditation facilitates detachment from the situation so the mind remains undisturbed. Without the stress and anxiety that might otherwise arise, it is possible to maintain a clear vision and see the Tao in the moment and understand the situation for what it is. With clear vision, it is easier to respond to the situation in the correct way. Thus, flexibility is maintained and each situation can be treated as fresh and new. In this way, being tied down to any hard and fast rules that the society imposes may be avoided. As a result, one does nothing that is unnatural or restrictive to the body and mind. Meditation frees us to get closer to our Tao.

Becoming a Taoist means becoming more realistic. Taoism respects and observes the uniqueness of the individual's nature instead of succumbing to human law or cultural norms. For centuries, Chinese governments have endorsed the Confucian philosophy as a human law. Historically, authorities have deemed Taoists a threat to their power because Taoists speak truth to power, potentially upsetting the current hierarchy.

We are only on this earth for a finite number of years. We must ask ourselves how we can make the best of it. Our happiness is not separate from others'. So, how can we make ourselves as well as others happy? We must help ourselves to help others. This means we must develop compassion. Essentially, compassion comes down to using the knowledge we gain for the benefit of others. This may include writing some of the insights and knowledge that we have for future generations — or simply living our lives well. We can leave positive footprints that contribute to the greater good of humanity in the world.

## 7.9
## What other benefits can be gained from this type of meditation?

Regular quiet sitting for periods of time allows a person's true nature to emerge. For example, someone might love to sketch but, because of family pressures, might become a physician instead of pursuing a career in the arts. However, in doing so, he is suppressing his nature or Tao. When his mind is clear and relaxed, however, he can make the correct choice. He can see what his path really is and follow it, rather than be miserable spending his life trying to please others by doing what they want him to do.

Another component of the meditation I teach is self-massage along the meridian points. The self-massage is practiced at the end of each meditation session. Meditation generates *chi*, which can pile up: so, to adjust the flow of *chi*, much like acupressure would, I teach students to massage themselves after each session. For more information, consult *Chu Meditation* (Chapter 6, "Self-Massage").

### 7.10
### Can you further elaborate on the benefits of Taoist meditation practice?

By practicing meditation, the mind becomes quiet and still while the body is relaxed. This neutral state of mind and body enhances flexibility and the ability to change stances at any moment, instead of being rigid and stuck. In other words, it improves overall sensitivity and responsiveness to all situations. Applied to fighting, when the opponent throws a punch, the appropriate response comes easily. We are so relaxed, actions seem slowed down to our eyes; and we can see the punch coming. We can be unafraid, respond beautifully, size up the situation correctly, and not overreact. This is the beginning step.

When one has achieved an advanced state in meditation, not only is response to another's action easier, it becomes possible to anticipate an opponent's intention and know what is coming. With this ability, things and events are seen "as they are" from both sides of a coin, so to speak. It is easy to see through the hypocrisy of politics, religions and other social standards. Their laws are artificial (as opposed to scientific or natural law). Largely, they exist only to benefit certain religious or political groups who will alter them whenever it is convenient to their own needs. It is important to remember there is a natural law of the universe, the Tao, that supercedes human laws. Human laws confine the uniqueness of the individual. The Taoist is involved with the society but not immersed to the extent that it hurts his or her Tao. Through meditation you gain "the ability to put yourself in a situation and take yourself out at will. Taoists call it *chu si* ('getting out') and *yup si* ('going in')" (*Chu Meditation*, p. 72). Detachment is very important so that you won't let a situation harm you. Mental strength is more powerful than physical strength, and meditation will give you such strength.

### 7.11
### In class, you mentioned that we develop "subconscious awareness" by practicing quiet sitting. What do you mean by this?

The body and mind have a built-in mechanism, an intrinsic awareness — this is "You," this is your "Tao." Due to cultural and religious customs and taboos, this intrinsic awareness is often suppressed. Then, it is nearly impossible to fulfill destiny or follow a path. For example, certain religions profess a belief in original sin and consider the natural act of sex unholy, dirty and sinful. However, the idea that humans are born sinners burdens the individual with guilt. Such logic affects the mind of the individual, and it also affects society negatively. Socially prescribed beliefs such as these can be difficult to erase from one's mind, and they may disturb one's intrinsic awareness and the health of society. Intrinsic awareness without interference helps us get back on the right path, so to speak. Take the sea turtle as an example. After birth, it drifts hundreds of miles away from its birthplace. Yet when it matures, it instinctively swims back to where it was born in order to lay eggs. If, however, the turtle is put under enough stress, it can lose touch with the intrinsic awareness that guides it on its natural path.

The relaxation that comes from doing tai chi and meditation lessens the constraints imposed by the rigidity of social and cultural systems, so that we can pursue the natural and positive vitality of the human species. As we free ourselves from social dogma, we become more in tune with our minds and bodies. Then, our intrinsic subconscious awareness emerges. This takes time. Nevertheless, as time passes, the degree of subconscious power will increase.

### 7.12
### How does one move the *chi* within the body: with the mind or will? Is this a dangerous practice?

The problem with moving *chi* with the mind is that an average person does not have enough *chi* to do it. In trying to do this, more energy will be wasted than gained. If the *chi* is strong from consistent meditation and *nei kung* over time, then the mind can move the *chi* easily. If the *chi* is low, the practice will do more harm than good.

### 7.13
### How can quietness be achieved in the city where it is noisy and hectic?

Practice correctly and consistently and you will achieve quietness, despite living amidst the noise of a city like New York.

All Taoist achievements require an inward development, which depends upon internal quietness. Quietness or *jing*, in Chinese, means there are no distractions. External stimuli must be shut out and the "monkey mind" (the incessant internal chattering that occurs in all of us) must be silenced. However, as with learning tai chi (which you cannot do correctly right away), a beginner cannot silence the mind right away — even if walled up in silent seclusion. It takes time. In the meditation I teach, the eyes are kept partially closed, to *decrease* sensory input. Through my technique, you steadily quiet the monkey mind over time.

For a beginner, earplugs and an eyeshade may be helpful. You may also need to habituate yourself to not reacting when disturbing noises arise, provided you are certain of being in a safe, secure environment. Tell yourself, "nothing bothers me," and don't give in to irritation or anger when a buzz saw comes on or car alarm goes off. If you cannot trust that noises will not distract you, use white noise. At a higher level, these aids will not be needed. In fact, with practice over a long time, the eyes can remain closed or open during meditation but not cause distraction. But for training, the majority of people need literally to close their senses to external feelings and let the body go inward a little bit. For this, aids may help.

Then the goal is to empty the mind, sometimes by counting slowly from one to ten or doing deep breathing, so that little by little the mind quiets down. The mind's focus narrows to something simple, for example, to the *tan tien* area. By narrowing the mind's focus to the *tan tien*, the energy and *chi* will be stronger. For the first few years of practice, "narrowing the mind" will not mean you are not thinking of other things at all. Rather, steadily, you think of those other things less and less. This happens because you can narrow the mind to whatever step of my meditation technique you are working on at that moment (see *Chu Meditation*).

The function of meditation is twofold: one, narrow the mind's thoughts and achieve quietness; two, achieve an energy-charging effect, rejuvenating the body. The *tan tien* is like a battery in an electrical system; when the mind is focused on it, energy is put into it, which can be stored and used later on. In meditation, instead of wasting energy by thinking about things, you recycle that energy and use it to charge the body up.

### 7.14
### Meditation seems easy. A person is just sitting there doing nothing. Should we learn meditation first, before learning *Eternal Spring*, tai chi or *nei kung*?

Meditation is one phase of tai chi training at CK Chu Tai Chi. According to my curriculum, a student first learns *Eternal Spring Chi Kung*, then tai chi, then *nei kung*, and, after that, the tai chi fast form. Only then does a student learn meditation.

Meditation can be very difficult for a total beginner. Sitting still is very challenging, both physically and mentally. The knees and back will ache and the mind will wander. All this hinders prolonged sitting. This is why it is better to begin meditation after achieving the level of patience and physical fitness that only comes with *Eternal Spring* and the other kinds of training. That is why at CK Chu Tai Chi, students are rarely allowed to start learning meditation right away.

On the other hand, meditation cannot be left out of training. The four areas of tai chi training, *chi kung*, tai chi forms and *nei kung*, and meditation, complement each other. In fact, to achieve a high level in these disciplines depends on doing a lot meditation. The four together harmonize the mind and body, which is the long-term goal.

The best way of learning anything is to work step by step, following a curriculum. People who want to jump around quickly just to learn more things will never achieve their goals. Meditation sounds simple and good — and no doubt, it is — but it is not simple to learn and is not an end in itself.

Besides, people already sit too much these days at computers or watching TV. In the old days, people in general were more active. Today, with sitting so much, people don't need extra sitting until they are really ready to learn to meditate. For this reason I suggest people come to the school and follow the curriculum. You will enjoy every moment of it, and when you start getting benefits you will never give it up.

**7.15**
### Does thinking use up a lot of energy?

Thinking, like any activity, uses up energy, but negative thinking drains the body more than even physical work. If you do a lot of physical activity, your body will get tired and you will fall asleep. However, if you are thinking and worrying too much, you can't fall asleep. Your system is not relaxed and your flow of *chi* is blocked. In certain cases, fearful and anxious thoughts can even short-circuit the system.

**7.16**
### What does it mean to short-circuit the system?

Think of the body's *chi* as an electrical system. All the body's activities require *chi* (electricity or energy). The mind needs more *chi* than the other systems, even the muscles when doing exercise. The mind is the central control system. Using the mind affects the body as a whole, the organs, the nervous system, etc. Thinking negative thoughts, like fear, stress, worry, and anxiety, is activity done by the mind that accomplishes nothing except dissipating *chi*. The more you do this type of negative thinking, the more *chi* is wasted. That energy could have gone to healing your body, purposive thinking, or bolstering your immune system; but instead, the negative thinking increases susceptibility to illnesses like ulcers and cancer. Disease is like a malfunction that results when the body is confused. In this case, negative thinking done in excess over a long period of time will affect the whole body. In my opinion, some cancers are the result of such long-term negative thinking. I think that negative thinking, more than genes and the environment, cause cancer. The power of the mind and its control in the body should not be underestimated. If the flow of energy throughout the whole body is disabled from constant worrying, problems will occur for the whole body. People need rest, they need to meditate, and they need to think positive thoughts. Positive thoughts relax and ease the system's *chi* flow.

**7.17**
### Does positive thinking drain the body?

Positive thinking means you are optimistic and relaxed. It does use some energy to think this way, but the body can recuperate from it quite easily. Positive thinking is fine and does not short-circuit the system.

**7.18**
### How long does it take before someone experiences *chi* during meditation?

An average person who is relaxed and healthy should feel the *chi* in a few months to a year, possibly even during a first meditation class. The sensation of warmth, in the face or hands — that's *chi*. It's the *chi* that makes you warm. However, achieving a high level as a meditation student and feeling *chi* in the *tan tien* area will take a few years.

### 7.19
### Can you describe some examples of feeling *chi*?

Sitting in meditation for at least a half an hour or so, should produce a sensation of heat going to your face. It will feel itchy, like ants crawling on your skin. That sensation is *chi* going through the meridians in your face. Any time you feel a tingling sensation of warmth in any part of the body, that's *chi*.

*Chi* is analogous to an electromagnetic wave — it is like a microwave. Food heats up in a microwave oven because the microwaves excite the food's water molecules. Your *chi* is like a microwave and warms up the water molecules in your system (see question 2.4). Heat signals that *chi* is flowing.

A high-level practitioner has strong *chi* in the *tan tien* and will actually feel *chi* shooting up from the base of his spine. But that takes a few years.

### 7.20
### Do you feel *chi* along the meridians?

The *chi* always goes through the meridians. Meridians are like wires carrying electricity. Some wires are bigger and can carry more current, and some are thinner and can carry less. The biggest meridian is from the *tan tien*, up the back to the top of the head and then down the front of the body in a big loop. This is called the *da chou tien*, meaning Big Orbit or Big Revolution. There are smaller meridians in the face.

### 7.21
### While meditating, is it correct to visualize the *chi* going through the body?

It is incorrect to try to visualize *chi* while doing tai chi (see 5.12), and this is also true for meditation. It is important to stop thinking and worrying while meditating. That is what makes the *chi* strong. If you visualize the *chi* in the meridians you will use up a lot of brain energy just to feel the little *chi* you have.

By visualizing, which is thinking, you are not charging up the *chi*; you are just feeling it. I repeat — ceasing to think makes the *chi* strong. Too much thinking and trying to feel the *chi* will drain the system. You might even end up short-circuiting it and getting a headache. Visualizing the *chi* does more harm than good.

### 7.22
### Should we try to move the *chi* throughout the body?

There are many steps of training before you should do this. The first step is to make the *chi* strong with sitting meditation and *nei kung*. When the *chi* is strong you will feel so much heat it will be like a radiator is next to you. This first step could take years and years of regular practice. Only then should you consider moving the *chi* through the body.

### 7.23
### Besides improving *chi*, what are the benefits of meditation?

I think one of the most important benefits of meditation and silence is that you will discover yourself, who you are, and how you fit into society. Society has many restrictions. You are not free to do whatever you want. You can't run in the street naked. You can't always speak freely. There are so many things you can't do, so really, you are not that free at all. Thus it is important to know your uniqueness and use this uniqueness to prosper in this restrained society. The first step in discovering yourself by consistent meditation is not easy. The next step of implementing or acting upon your discovery of yourself is even more difficult. You need a lot of self-discipline to accomplish this goal. Fortunately, meditation unleashes your power to know yourself.

### 7.24
### Is there any other step I can take to achieve quietness (*jing*)?

Yes. There are two major qualities we can incorporate in our lives: *ching* which means purity and simplicity, and *ding* which means steadiness.

*Ching* is like a sky with no clouds in it — simple, pure. Sometimes the word is used alongside *jing*, like *ching-jing*, to mean simple, clear, uncomplicated and quiet. To achieve *jing*, sometimes one may have to acquire *ching* first. To have *ching* means to simplify our life, to be more selective about our activities.

Modern society in general is not too *ching*. In a city like New York, just to understand the telephone bill we need a doctorate in telephone-bill-paying. Our society is the opposite of *ching*: very, very complex. So to develop *ching*, the first step is to *clear stuff away*. Take clothing, for example: there are winter clothes, summer clothes, this style, that style — it drives you crazy. So, how can you develop *ching*? In terms of clothing, just wear something simple. It is far more important to wear clothes that are functional, healthy and clean than to be victim of trends and fads. Taoists do not really care about fashion; instead, they are more concerned with essentials: nutrition, clean air, a healthy mind, less noise pollution, a more natural lifestyle.

Somebody may have the best clothing there is, but we can see in his or her face, in the quality of the skin or the eyes, or in the smell of the toxins in the sweat, that internally they are not healthy; perfume and make-up cannot cover that up. To attain *ching* requires more internal work. We must simplify our lives internally in order to simplify our lives externally.

So, *jing* and *ching* are linked together. *Ching*, *jing*, and *ding*. *Ding* is the quality of steadiness. *Ding* means we have an even temperament, no turbulence. That is why if we go to any temple or place of worship, the first thing we notice is that it is simple and quiet. The body actually needs that sometimes. Of course, sometimes the body wants a lot of activity. But most of the time, the body wants *jing*.

When people do not have enough *jing* and *ching*, they go crazy. With too much noise pollution, media pollution, they do not have a chance to be themselves. So what do they do? They smoke, they drink alcohol and coffee, and all these things will affect the mind. They follow what advertisers tell them about smoking and drinking, and, like a rat in an experiment that is overfed a substance, they may make poor decisions.

The opposite frame of mind is *ching-jing*: through quietness comes clarity and better decision-making. When a person makes good decisions, it is not only good for him but for the whole society. And, on the other hand, if many people give off bad vibes, everybody who comes in contact with them, physically or even through electronic media, will be affected. We could say *jing* and *ching* is the essence or the beginning of Taoist self-cultivation.

### 7.25
### Why does emptying the mind feel terrifying, like a little "death"?

When the mind is empty of thoughts, that means we are unconscious. We do not know what is going on: it is like being soundly asleep. It is common for fear and paranoia to emerge when we enter this state of emptiness. Most of us were raised with stories about ghosts and spirits. These ghosts, spirits and monsters exist in our minds on the subconscious level. When we sit quietly, our subconscious fear of these things begins to surface.

For many years as a child, I was afraid of the dark because I thought a ghost would appear. It wasn't until much later that I realized that no such things existed. Spirits of the dead are scientifically impossible phenomena. At least this is what I believe. Once I realized this, my fear of darkness disappeared. That is my story; people can have different kinds of phobias.

In the Chu Meditation method, emptying the mind is not the first step. As we learn to meditate, we focus on one narrow theme at a time. We start with Step 1: Head Suspended, then move on to the next step, then the next. The mind is working. We are meditating, and not yet empty. Not until Step 4, in which we count numbers over and over, does the mind slowly start to drift off to emptiness. If one follows the procedure, one will not give ghosts and spirits or fears a chance to sneak into one's mind while sitting. When we are alone, we can become fearful of emptiness or death as the mind thinks about everything, especially things that bother us. That is why one needs this method which keeps one's mind focused on a single task at a time. In each of the 5 steps, as soon as you find your mind wandering or thinking about fearful things, you should bring it back to the task of "Mind to the *Tan Tien*," or "Head Suspended," etc. This is how one empties one's mind without entering the stage of fearfulness. Many people the world over still believe in ghosts and spirits. While these beliefs will not be discarded any time soon, the Chu Meditation method will help us keep our heads in the right place.

# VIII. TAI CHI AND SEX

## 8.1
## What is the Taoist view on sex?

The Chinese word "Tao" means "the way." To the Taoist, Tao is synonymous with science, as it adheres to a scientific way of exploring life. As suggested earlier in this text, approaching life scientifically, or in a Taoist fashion, means there is a natural path for phenomena to follow and any attempt to work against or obstruct this path will lead to social problems or disease. Trees have a cycle, as does the earth. Humans can study the Tao of the trees or the earth to help, or hinder, trees and the earth on their path. For humans, the natural path is to be born a baby, grow up, become an adolescent, have sex, raise children, grow old, become weak, and die. Humans have a natural cycle: sex is part of that cycle and should therefore be accepted — not obstructed with laws and taboos. Even Confucius, who embraces many social attitudes that oppose those of the Taoist's, unequivocally agrees on this subject. He says, "eating and sex are human nature." "Nature" means it is the natural law and human law should not interfere with that. To both Taoists and Confucians, there is no question that everyone needs good food and sex. Anything that contradicts or denies such basic human needs would not be natural, hence not Taoist. It would be going against life and nature itself, leading to negative repercussions.

## 8.2
## How does tai chi affect sex?

We gain much from tai chi. When we practice tai chi, the body is more relaxed and the mind is calmer. We become more aware, and as our awareness increases, we're more attuned to our body. Our body and mind both become strong yet flexible. To have good sex, one needs to be strong and flexible, as well as responsive to his or her partner. Practicing tai chi increases sexual energy by developing strong *chi* and charging up the body. Good sex is actually good physical exercise. When you do tai chi, you increase your overall fitness and, specifically, the range of motion. It is like a bonus for performing good sex because you make the joints, lower back, and especially the knees, stronger, and your mind is relaxed and tuned into the activity. Doing tai chi correctly will increase vitality and youthfulness.

Many people experience tiredness after sex because their body is too rigid and the mind is not relaxed; so, the sex act just drains energy. This makes them exhausted, because this physical act puts demands on certain parts of the body. Tai chi and *nei kung* can revitalize the body. Sex is about two partners successfully linking together, physically and mentally. It's about relating and responding to each other well. It's not a one-way street. Good sex is a result of good integration between two people. It's the *yin* and the *yang* completing one whole circle. One's body has to be in good shape, which tai chi develops, to have good sex.

### 8.3
### What do fighting arts have to do with sex?

The most important part of fighting is responding. Tai chi trains you to respond through push-hands exercise. In tai chi we practice push-hands to learn how to sense the opponent's attacking power and energy, and redirect it in order to overcome him. Optimal sex is like push-hands. You've got to get a sense of your partner — what he or she wants and what you want. One has to feel the partner's energy, respond to it, and this goes back and forth, from low-level responding to high-level responding. When you are relaxed, the feeling will move you. The continuation of responding will lead you to the highest relaxation and pleasurable feelings and that will lead to the highest climax.

For example, it has been documented that the turtle has great longevity. One of the reasons may be that turtles are relaxed and enjoy sex. They do it slowly and enjoy sex for days. People can't have sex for days, but, when relaxed, people should be able to have sex for hours. The longer sex lasts, the better the sperm and eggs. A healthy couple should be able to have sex for two to eight hours. When this happens, this is good sex. Having sex for a long time stimulates the body and, for men, makes the sperm strong and healthy. That is why if you plan to have a baby, it is important for men not to climax too soon. A healthy sex life makes for healthy children because healthy sex, or optimal sex, takes place between two people who are in good shape — mentally, physically, and spiritually. Before conceiving a child, these two healthy people will have first formed sound preliminary emotional and physical connections that establish a positive energy between them. The woman will have healthy, viable eggs. The man will have healthy, viable sperm. Then, during the sex act itself, the couple will warm up the bodies appropriately achieving a positively charged connection and then their healthy egg and healthy sperm will come together due to a good sexual experience. The baby born as a result will be healthy and happy.

Tai chi practice, and especially *nei kung*, charges up the body so that one is full of energy. Even an older person can feel like a teenager. In fighting, we use our ability to respond to any situation to overcome our opponent. In sex, we use our sensitivity to respond to our partner's needs. Just like you need good food, you need good sex. Good sex makes people healthy and young.

## 8.4
## Is sex good for health?

Sex is an exercise in which the body moves in certain ways — stretching, opening and bending. The muscles, tendons and even the bones can develop through it. Tai chi, *chi kung*, and *nei kung* develop the body in similar ways. If one cannot stretch and bend his or her knees well, one cannot have good sex. If performed correctly, sex is a good exercise. In addition to strengthening the muscles, tendons and bones, it also stimulates the body and the mind. It increases blood and *chi* circulation and stimulates the heart, the lungs, and all other internal organs. Sex maintains one's physical functions. And just like any good exercise, recuperation time is needed after sex. If one does not have sex, the body, the *chi* and the internal organs are probably not functioning optimally. With no sex or bad sex, our body can become stiff and our mind full of negativity. By bad sex I mean sex that is forced, tensed (body unhealthy, mind not at ease), rushed, yields no satisfaction, unnatural, or is negatively charged in any way. With good sexual energy the body is more relaxed, and the mind is more positive. This, in turn, helps you realize your life potential or Tao.

## 8.5
## Can sex without release increase the body's *chi*?

The answer is yes, but you have to do it naturally and with a relaxed mind. It cannot be forced. Then sex becomes like high-level *chi kung*, an exercise that increases the body's *chi*. But this does not mean you should never release. Never releasing is not natural.

Taoism teaches that humans have what is called *intrinsic ching*, which, in men, can become *chi* or *common ching* (sperm). For a man, release during sex means losing a certain amount of his sexual energy or *ching*, which can lead to tiredness and irritability.

This requires correct application of specific nutrition and rest, which could be tricky. So, sex without release and the subsequent draining of energy is correct practice according to Taoist teachings.

The question about how often a man should release depends on the individual and often his age. He can release more often when he's younger and less as he becomes older. If he's sexually active, he can determine his own rhythm by paying attention to his feelings the day after having sex. If he feels mostly fine, he's doing 'OK.' But if he feels overly tired or experiences negative emotions, he probably needs to release less often.

### 8.6
### I thought Taoist monks practice celibacy.

There are numerous branches of Taoism today. As far as I know, outside of Christianity, only Buddhist monks promote celibacy. Taoist priests are allowed to have sex. In fact, some Taoist priests encourage older men to engage in more sexual activities without frequent release. I find celibacy problematic because sexual release is a natural function of the body. Men should release at least once in a while. It is just like a dam that controls the flow of the river. The water in the reservoir needs to be released periodically or it will overflow. Complete celibacy means the flowing water is dammed up unnaturally. When the sexual organs are not used, this negatively affects the rest of the body. For that reason, among others, I have reservations about it. It is one thing to control release, but another to suppress it completely. Negative repercussions will surely follow.

Celibacy is a manmade discipline; it is not natural. Too much of anything is no good, no matter what it is. The answer is moderation and discipline. This discipline should not be forced. For Taoists, discipline is like a dam; it's used to control the flow of water but not to stop it. Building a dam is constructive; it's analogous to saving money in the sense that one has more money to spend on bigger projects later (like more sperm with which to conceive a child).

### 8.7
### Why are religions so obsessed with sex?

I don't know why organized religions are against sex. The only reason I can think of is because when you have sex you are more relaxed. When you are relaxed you are following your Tao (natural law). Many religious beliefs are against natural law. They have stories and fairy tales that are the same as believing in Santa Claus.

To be a Taoist means to approach life scientifically. Religions are human-made. They are not divine. Religious organizations are corporations with their own agenda, which often involve self-promotion. Taoists try to free themselves from religion. This is, of course, not easy if you are brought up with these traditions. The influence of religion might take forever to shake off, but it is worth trying.

### 8.8
### What is your opinion about sex in a civilized society?

We think we are "civilized" but according to the Taoist view of sex, animals are more civilized than we are. They do the act of sex but don't have the taboos we have. We are, of course, more intelligent than they are but they are closer to Tao. We have too many problems about sex in our culture. In other words, we try to have the human law supercede the natural law. Just because we dress in clothing and have technology does not make us civilized.

## 8.9
## What would make us civilized with regard to sex?

Sex is like food. People need it; there should be no law against it, period. Suppression of nature creates problems and myths. Otherwise, without suppression, sex would be normal. Go to a restaurant and have good food and then go have good sex.

If people have good sex, that means they are healthy; their body is functioning well and they can reproduce. Sex and health are linked together. If you are healthy, you have more sex drive. Good sex leads to higher sperm count and that leads to healthier babies. In turn, the species, the whole of human civilization, is stronger. Ideally you should have a lot of education about what to eat, what makes good sex and how to have it. Schools do not teach such things and you see the results — runaway obesity and suppressed sex drives and other problems.

In general, people should not judge others. Criminalizing sex, educating people to detest sex, and encouraging bad sex prevent millions of people from being natural, being true to their Tao, and thus they live unbalanced and unhealthy lives. Such a negative attitude toward sex is strange to me. It is as if people who detest sex want problems in society and want unhealthy babies in the future. When people eat incorrectly and have a health problem as a result, they get mad and want drugs to allow them to continue eating incorrectly. Likewise, bad sex and the consideration of sex as impure or sinful has to be rethought. First, this negative approach to sex affects the mind, burdening it with negativity and stress. Second, such negativity affects the body, since sex is not the healthy activity it should be. Thinking that sex is obscene throws you off and adds an unnecessary constraint on your system. The whole morality of sex, whether it is legal or criminal, creates a negative approach to sex that can cause disease. People have difficulty talking about the link between poor health in the population and bad eating habits, but at least there is some discussion. Unfortunately, people don't even think about the link between good health and good sex. People should be happy and that depends on eating healthily, exercising, and having good sex.

## 8.10
## What does marriage have to do with sex?

Marriage is a legal contract in society that is concerned with matters of property ownership and the inheritance of property. It has nothing to do with sex and people should remind themselves of this fact. Marriage also exists to try to create a formal society but, in my opinion, it can create a lot of problems. In that sense, sometimes marriage is useful and sometimes it is not useful. We must remember that marriage and sex are two different phenomena. We should not tie sex to marriage.

### 8.11
### Do you support sex education in schools?

Yes. The lack of correct sex education or sex education at all, is a major problem. Part of education's purpose is to dispel the myths and fables of yesterday and to provide children with the tools they need for a better, healthier tomorrow. But too many parents, teachers, and politicians are themselves confused about sex. They see it through the eyes of organized religion, which views sex as shameful — however necessary. They simply don't want their children to have any exposure to this topic. Thus the circle continues and the children of people who fear sex will, consequently, fear sex. Correctly, sex should enable people to know one another better. It is a loving act. Education should teach it this way.

Sex education must be scientific. It also must cover such basic facts as sexual hygiene. Misunderstandings about sex can needlessly lead to the spread of disease.

This would be better than sex education being viewed as embarrassing and a topic to be kept in the closet. In fact, in the old days in China, they actually had people teach sex. Before getting married, an older person would teach and coach the young people. Young people should receive good information about sex as well as about physical fitness and nutrition. To me, the current state of sex education is like something from the Dark Ages and it is completely non-scientific.

### 8.12
### What happens when we suppress sexual energy?

If you go into an ocean with a beach ball and press the ball underwater, the deeper and deeper you push, the more force you'll need to keep the ball down. After a certain point you can't push it any further and the ball must pop up; and the deeper you've pushed the ball, the higher it will pop up.

The same is true when you suppress sex. You can try to deny your natural sexual impulses, but after a certain point you will have to channel them somewhere. And the longer you deny the natural aspect of sex, the more these impulses will have a negative and destructive effect on both your sex life and your life as a whole.

Think of a flowing river. Sexual energy flows down the same way water goes downhill. When you suppress the water, it will flow in a different direction. It will have to go somewhere. For men, the sperm needs to go somewhere, so it will. And it may go haywire and flood to places you don't want it to. That's why there are cases of celibate clergy committing molestation and pedophilia: their suppressed sexual energy was eventually expressed in a most harmful way.

As human beings, we have natural urges and repressing those urges negatively affects our emotions and our self-control. Repression results from misguided self-control (for example, after being dumped by a significant other, you swear off all sex), religious law (which regards sex as something shameful), or state law (which criminalizes certain sex acts due to cultural prohibitions). Whatever the reason for repression in the first place, buying into the idea that sex is a sin is also a condemnation of yourself — of who you are as a human being. The consequences of such self-condemnation, and, by extension, the condemnation of others, can be bad. While everyone is different, repressed sexual energy in some people may be misdirected into crime or violence against a spouse, a child, or someone else.

Even when it doesn't lead to acts of violence, this perspective on sex makes you ashamed and susceptible to manipulation. This makes for a corrupt society. Take the fight over gay sex and gay marriage. Homosexuals are human beings and condemning them due to religious notions of what is or is not a proper sex act has created huge problems. On the one hand, people are denied rights; on the other hand, the loudest voices condemning homosexuality originate in people who turn out to be self-hating homosexuals. By buying into the idea that sex is shameful, they first condemned themselves and then others while helping to create a negativity in society that became manifest in inhumane laws.

### 8.13
### What about people who consider sex obscene?

I'm always amazed that in this society people use a sex word as a curse word. Our culture has become warped through religion and centuries of taboo against women. We consider "F U!" as a way to hurt someone, when actually "F U!" is not violent or a curse. It is only a curse because of a cultural problem. "F U" is the act of love. It is constructive.

If you go to a movie you cannot see a natural sex act or people talking like adults, but you can see people graphically hurting and gruesomely torturing one another. This is a major problem and reminds me that many people who are against sex are for war. There seems to be an association there. That's why in the 1960's we would say, "make love not war." Sex is positive, not negative.

### 8.14
### What about violence and sex?

We confuse sex with violence because of repression. If you cannot have regular sex, you have no normal outlet for those desires. War, rape, and other out-of-control situations are perpetrated largely by people who don't have a healthy outlet for their sexual energy. To overcome this problem, we should have positive, constructive sex. That should be a priority in terms of civilized society. A civilized society should be measured by how people treat sex. Scandinavian society is considered to be more open about sex and, as far as I'm concerned, is therefore more civilized.

## 8.15
## How can the average person benefit from your teaching regarding sex?

Sex is part of healthy, positive living. By doing tai chi, *chi kung*, *nei kung*, and meditation, the body and the mind achieve their best state of being, composing a well rounded person — the best you. In such a state, there is more energy for sex, which is simply a biological function. Now, whether you are able to find a partner with the same views is another story. She or he may be wrapped up in the myths and the negative, violent attitudes toward sex all too prevalent in society. Worse, he or she is probably not aware of harboring negative views of sex. It is not true to Taoism to try and convert your partner in any way, but if he or she is willing to discuss sex, you should talk about it openly and freely.

So the answer is: make yourself the best you can be and the sex you then have will be more enjoyable. If possible, find sex partners who are, like you, being the best they can be. That is the difficult part. A person you like may not match you because of their attitude to sex. That is unfortunate. Perhaps, with more sex education, future humans will be more open about it and have better sex. This will lead to a healthy society and better offspring. Better sex, like a better body and a better world, is a long-term project. It takes time to convince people to change. You may have to look hard for this person since you cannot force someone to re-examine his or her views of sex. Put it this way: we are all influenced by negative attitudes towards sex in this society and this is definitely not good. But if you are in pursuit of your Tao, you will have a healthier attitude towards sex and that may be enough to help your partner do the same.

# IX. TAI CHI IN DAILY LIFE

## 9.1
## What impact can tai chi have on daily life?

Besides being an art of self-defense, tai chi is an art of life. Aside from the improvements in physical and mental health, those who practice tai chi live a tai chi way of life. The core principle of tai chi is *yin* and *yang*. When an opponent attacks you with a strong *yang* force, you use a *yin* force to yield because your opponent might be too strong for you to be able to use your force against his force. Tai chi teaches you to overcome a stronger opponent using the principle that four ounces overcomes one thousand pounds of force.

Yielding in tai chi is analogous to the way a matador fights a bull. The one thousand pound bull charges the matador, and the closer the matador is to the bull, the more effective he is in returning the attack.

This same principle can be applied in daily life. Suppose you are working a job and your boss is very aggressive. You can't fight your boss using force against force. You must yield and tell your boss he is right while still proposing another solution. Telling him he's wrong directly may get you fired. Instead, by engaging and yielding, depending on the situation, you can come out ahead. Maybe your boss will listen to you and something constructive can happen. That is using tai chi principles in daily life.

## 9.2
## Can this yielding apply to any situation?

Absolutely. Tai chi yielding means you are not rigid. You are flexible and able to overcome any situation. As challenges arise, you learn how to assess them to come up with options for response. Then, you select the best response for you but you know there may be a learning curve, as they say. If you don't succeed the first time, obviously you must try again and again until you find a solution that works. Trying again means you are flexible.

Tai Chi yielding means going with the flow. Think of tall dune grass on a beach. No matter how strong the wind is, the tall grass bends and bounces back. We don't want to be like an old tree — dried up and rigid so that when the wind comes, the tree cracks and collapses. Yielding means repositioning at all times to your advantage as if in a game of chess. You try your best to checkmate your opponent so that you are in control of the game. Likewise in life, you must checkmate whatever decision you have to make by yielding so as to reposition yourself into control of the situation.

### 9.3
### How do I yield my way into a better job?

It is important to assess any job. See if it is suited to you and if it's what you really want to do. Of course, if you cannot get the job you want, you have no choice but to take some other job to pay your living expenses. You must do this other job while still searching for one better suited to your Tao.

There is an old Chinese expression, "Riding a water buffalo while looking for a horse." This means that you shouldn't just walk around looking for a horse. Ride the water buffalo in the meantime. This approach is more realistic and more flexible.

### 9.4
### What if I look for a long time and still can't get a job I want?

Two things come to mind — patience and discipline. I think these two qualities are very important. Both are easier said than done, and few people have either. Having the patience to look for a job and the discipline to try to get it requires practice and training. It is not easy but it is worth trying.

In terms of cultivating your own Tao, little material wealth is required. Anyone can get a "job," although perhaps not one to your liking (and ideally your job will align with your Tao), but any job can be used to finance the activities you are interested in. If you cannot find a job, you can create your own. It may be that you do not yet understand yourself well enough, and you need to meditate more until what you really want in life becomes clear. Get a job to survive that does not require commitment — just something to get the pay you need to support yourself. If you have unrealistically high expectations, you may be disappointed and frustrated — that is not finding your Tao. You have to be realistic about the need to pay the rent and so on.

If you like to sing but are not able to make money from singing to pay your expenses, you must resort to singing as a hobby. You may end up riding the buffalo longer than you thought but you will learn to be happy, finding the time to do your own thing.

The question raises another set of issues. In American society, most people desire more money through a better "job" and look at their current job as temporary, instead of being engaged in a lifetime vocation. This is actually a cause of the current crisis (a similar culture of impermanence has resulted in the marred landscape of suburban sprawl). With everyone looking to get a better-paying job, hardly anybody tried to do their work in a manner responsible to the community. People just sought the fastest buck — bankers sold bad loans knowing they would default. In capitalism, the way to become filthy rich is to exploit other people and the earth. Our current economy was built on the hollow promise of the "American Dream" — get rich by doing nothing. A society promising that everyone can get rich by doing nothing is headed for trouble. Now, I imagine and hope, there will be a restructuring of the economy both by individuals and by institutions. The pursuit of the "fast buck" is not the game of the Taoist but of the con artist.

There may seem to be a contradiction here but my point is that in this world, dominated as it is by a "fast buck" mentality, we need to survive while improving ourselves so we can improve the world.

The *Tao Te Ching* describes wealth and richness in terms of contentment rather than money. The "American Dream" is the "Cinderella" myth: you happen to get lucky and the Prince likes you, no work required. But this "American Dream" can never be realized since it happens or it doesn't, and if it does, you still won't find contentment. Whether you are super-rich or super-poor, you are still poor if you are not content. It's hard to say which is worse, but in both, you lack contentment. If you are not content, you are not rich. As long as you are content you are "rich," and will be happier than most people — especially somebody who has to hold an unpleasant job to survive. Contentment is being healthy in body, sound in mind, aware of your own Tao, and living a purposeful life.

### 9.5
### If I practice tai chi, will I really see progress in other areas of my life?

Certainly. You will be healthier, calmer and see things more clearly. You will be able to formulate questions about your life and answer them. Most people can't even formulate questions about what they want, never mind trying to figure out how to get what they want. If you practice tai chi and meditation, you will be able to discover what you want in life and thus be able to pursue it better. Tai chi helps you discover your unique point of view.

### 9.6
### What can I study to round out a quality tai chi lifestyle?

I would say if you study tai chi without understanding the philosophical underpinnings of Taoism, it is only a physical act. If you want to go to a deeper level, beyond the mechanics of how to move the body, it is essential to learn Taoist philosophy, which supports your efforts to harmonize with nature and operate in connection with the essence of life.

Read more about Taoist philosophy — especially the *Tao Te Ching*. Unfortunately, most translations of the *Tao Te Ching* have problems. Many of the concepts are misinterpreted because the translator does not have a background in Taoism and tai chi or even speak or read Chinese. This is why I am planning to translate the book as I see it. This project may take a few years.

### 9.7
### Do you think that tai chi and meditation can resolve world issues?

The answer is definitely yes, but we face an uphill battle against many organized powers, as you could call them, which have become structural elements in our society. By doing tai chi and practicing meditation, as discussed throughout this book, people become healthier in mind and body. A healthy person is happier and less likely to experience or spread the negativity that causes conflict or problems. Through mental cultivation, healthy people come to see themselves and the world more clearly. They will see what is actually needed and what is not: what is important and what is not. Such a person will pursue the Tao, that which is natural and correct. Many people pursuing the Tao will result in a society without organization or power structures, but consisting of people using knowledge and reason to solve the problems of the moment. Given the number of people interested in meditation, tai chi, and self-improvement, there is reason to hope for a better future. Yet, as I said, one must acknowledge the steepness of the climb. The world's current problems result from the inertia of history. Solutions will come only through education and self-cultivation by everyone over time.

So, the more people who are Taoists or the more Taoist people become, the more decisions, at the personal and societal level, will be made according to the needs of individuals, rather than organized powers. Then society will be human-focused (whereas now, American society is property-focused). In a future book, I hope to expand on what Taoism can contribute to the renewal of humanity and of the earth on which we live.

### 9.8
### Can you give specific examples of the type of "organized powers" that stand in the way of a more humane and more reasoned society?

There is a long list of these powers, as far as I am concerned, but I think there are three big ones. If these three are faced — and that will require drastic action — then the world will be changed dramatically. These three are: organized religion, the military-industrial-university-congressional-complex, and organized crime. Power corrupts individuals and society and these three powers are at the root of the world's problems, environmental and social, because they prevent people from seeing clearly and acting rationally. These organized powers will want their power to continue and expand. It will be very hard to get rid of them...

### 9.9
### I understand that you plan on explaining how Taoism can help in a future book, could you just briefly explain how these powers stymie social progress?

Though the days of the Inquisition are long gone, organized religion still stymies rational inquiry and science. Western religions claim to have the absolute truth and their followers, like soldiers, confess that truth and cease to cultivate their understanding of both "spiritual" and "worldly" matters. Religion, especially in the US, continues to propagate ideas long dismissed elsewhere in the world, like "creationism," recently re-branded as "intelligent design." People with money disseminate these tired ideas and those with weak minds accept them. Reactivating creationism has made it almost impossible to have a sound science curriculum in the grade schools in the U.S. Worse, that type of belief system travels with the idea that God gave the earth to humans to use and abuse — the so-called "Wise Use" ideology. Thus, meaningful discussions of issues in science, including global climate change, are very difficult to have in the U.S. Since the people and their representatives cannot have this conversation, policy is being made by organized powers. Corporations, especially those involved in energy production, not only fund the confusion about climate change amongst the electorate, but they then pay lobbyists and make campaign contributions so that energy policy is made to serve their interests, not the people's (remember the Energy Task Force formed at the start of the previous administration — the only non-governmental entities they consulted with were energy corporations). Consequently, corporations, not the voters, are setting policy.

The history of how corporations have gained their power is complicated and long. To my mind, the most significant moment came during WWII when corporations, which had been severely weakened by the Depression, regained their power through war profiteering. As corporations by definition exist to make money, they cannot be socially responsible. Instead, they do what they can to perpetuate war. Having come into power by winning WWII, they have increasingly centralized power ever since. It will be very difficult to redistribute power away from corporations, especially now after the decision in *Citizens United v. Federal Election Commission*, which found that corporate campaign contributions cannot be limited. One solution might be to make war profiteering illegal, for this would steer the profit seekers away from war.

Eisenhower first mentioned the dangers inherent in the military-industrial complex. The well-known term was shortened for effect but Eisenhower's speechwriters had also included the universities and the U.S. Congress in the "complex." Half a century later they have been proven correct. War is now endless as it serves the complex. Perpetual war results in the purchase of more weapons and owning weapons leads to the use of weapons. The US may have won WWII but it then spent $4 trillion fighting a Cold War. So while European countries rebuilt their countries, the U.S. spent its treasure on weapons. Imagine what the US would look like today if it had not made control of the world a priority. Once the Cold War was over, the complex tried to create a new enemy because without an enemy, weapons are not needed. First it tried China, then Iraq and Islam, and now it's an idea — Terrorism (which, as an idea, can never be defeated). It is not healthy to view the world in Manichean terms: "good v. evil" only leads to war, and it solves nothing. Universities are increasingly dependent on the research dollars attached to defense while any talk of trimming the Pentagon's budget always encounters the congressman convinced that his voters will wind up homeless if they cannot make bombs. What a waste of resources, making bombs.

The more laws there are, the more criminals there will be and the more criminality. Prohibition is the most famous example. Americans outlawed alcohol and created the romance of Al Capone. This was reversed to give people solace during the Depression and take away a source of disloyalty — even states know there are limits to laws. Most people must follow them: few followed Prohibition. President Nixon tried it again by launching the War on Drugs. The circumstances and substances were different but the outcome has been the same. What is the result? Even after an expenditure of one trillion dollars, the War on Drugs is a complete failure. Drugs are cheaper but of higher quality, while the cartels providing the drugs are stronger then ever. Decriminalize drugs and you stop wasting money, you eliminate the cartels, and drug use can be made safer for those who are going to use them anyway.

### 9.10
### So what would a more humane world look like?

Fewer moral laws and more regulation of the organized powers. Wall Street needs laws; people's sex lives do not. Most people are not strong enough to shake off the culture and religion they were born into; they cannot see beyond the prejudices of that culture or religion. Tai chi training makes the mind and body stronger so people can see more clearly.

The "Golden Rule" is a good idea; do we need any other moral rules? This topic requires more discussion than is possible here and it also requires meditation. However, when free of inherited or learned biases, humans the world over come to the same basic set of ideas. Look at those moments in history when people organized themselves, like the Paris Commune while it lasted. There, egalitarianism reigned, without hierarchy or dominance of any kind. Since organized religions create power structures, not personal happiness, they would be absent from such a world. Society should be classless and cooperation should be the rule; the fewer the laws, the better.

As I've said earlier in this book (see 8.14) the ideal society to me is Scandinavia. They have fewer laws there and the people are more liberal and more civilized. The uncivilized countries have more rules. The more rules, the more laws, the more taboos — the less civilized. Think of a country's so-called law and order: they make the laws and you take the orders.

## 9.11
## In what way does tai chi encompass a spiritual component?

Many people associate the word "spiritual" with God or gods, not our earthly lives. To me, the tai chi spiritual view means a person is very centered, understanding, logical, and scientific. You are able to connect with people and share their feelings. You understand people. Ideally, when you talk with people, their problems are your problems and you try to help them the best you can. If you can do that, it means you are confident in yourself and that nothing hinders you.

On the other hand, being non-spiritual means you undermine people and are preoccupied with gossip and mockery. You misinterpret the word "spiritual," and use it as an excuse to believe in the supernatural and to act "holier than thou." You judge people by your own narrow standards instead of trying to understand another's circumstances and background.

In general, our culture and society does not value people helping each other. It over-emphasizes too many artificial laws, which inhibit the mind and body. To me, being spiritual means being natural, which comes from within the Tao. It is dealing with everyday problems and the world's problems with the best logical and scientific mind and inner intuition — it comes from the heart. We are born with spirituality, but growing up, we become corrupted.

For example, we have an unnatural emphasis on ego, glory, and most of all, trivial competition — the idea that being first place is the only thing in the world that matters, and that when a guy gets second place, he should cry. From the perspective of the entire world, second place is not bad at all! Most trivial competition hurts progress. Instead, simply try your best and the Tao and tai chi philosophy will harmonize you with yourself and the environment. This gives you a view of the world that is both carefree and realistic. As the human race evolves, the positive energy of Tao philosophy will pull us out of our over-religious and cultural taboos laden lives.

Each culture has its own positive and negative traits; likewise, each person has positive and negative traits. Ideally, progress consists of identifying the positive traits and enhancing them while getting rid of the negative ones. To me, the people who do both, who work to improve themselves and society in this way, have attained the highest kind of spirituality.

Each human being is only here on earth for maybe a hundred years. Compared to the billions of years the universe has existed, we are only a spark that comes and goes. Appreciate life. Enjoy life. Do the best you can. Don't play the games people play. Spirituality should be natural and come from within. It should have nothing artificial about it, nothing to do with God and gods and angels or Santa Claus.

# AFTERWORD: THE TAO, THE WORLD, AND BEYOND

### *Wu Wei* — 'Let it be.'

The Chinese saying, *"wu wei,"* means doing something that seemingly does not lead to financial gain or career advancement. It does not promote you or earn you prestige. Tai chi is *wu wei*. It has the spirit of a hobby and does not involve striving for money or reputation. However, by following your body, you accomplish more than you realize and much more than by trying too hard and pursuing the vanity of society. That's what appeals to me about tai chi. It looks like I'm doing "nothing," yet I am gaining "everything." The idea of *wu wei* is exactly the idea in The Beatles' 1970 song "Let It Be." Paul McCartney captured a sense of *wu wei* in the phrase, 'let it be.' More *wu wei* would be very good for our world today.

It seems today that everyone is just out for money and material gain at the expense of others. People say they want to be a doctor or lawyer but not in order to help people. Instead, they assume those professions will make lots of money. However, if you have no actual interest in medicine or law, you will be wasting your time and trying too hard while accomplishing little. Chasing artificial goals makes life boring as hell. Society does not encourage people to be themselves and even fosters cynicism toward others. Our bourgeois society is structured so that a kid has to be competitive in kindergarten, continue struggling in elementary school, and all the way through college. This makes the body rigid and ruins the mind. I recall hearing Gore Vidal muse "that people at the age of six are very interesting, curious, and smart, but they are not interesting, curious, or smart, by the time they are sixteen." Something is wrong with our society and education system that allows this to happen.

Chasing school, jobs, money… that is not a life. There is more to life than making money just to stay alive. What kind of life is that anyway — just, money, eating and sleeping!? What a waste. Why not do something you are interested in? Pursue literature, science, art, or music. But no matter what you do, you need to maintain your body. Plus, how do you know what it is you want to do? You discover that by not trying so hard — just letting it be. Don't pigeonhole your life as "lawyer" so early for artificial reasons. Discover who you are by doing tai chi. That is the idea of *wu wei* — just doing it to do it, because you want to do it. So tai chi is training for life, training to discover the real you. We need more spontaneity. The progress of humanity comes through the people who do *wu wei* — not the ones that chase money. People think they have to know *what* they want. But *why*? I don't know what I want to be. Just let it, let yourself be. That is a typical idea of Taoism. You are like a child, always in an evolving stage of development. Flexible and not molded into something. You never want to be molded. The tool that keeps you 'yourself' both philosophically and mechanically is tai chi.

There is nothing worse than doing a job just because you have to. If you must dig ditches because someone commands you to, you will hate it. But if you dig ditches to help construct a project you love, you will enjoy it. Now, the same act has an entirely different meaning. The action looks the same, but physically and mentally it has a different outcome and feeling.

### It's Not Easy Though — So How Can This Be Achieved?

Unfortunately, in the world we usually have to do certain things we don't want to do.

By learning tai chi, you will hopefully have to do less and less of what you don't want to do. That is the beauty of tai chi and of life. Life is about evolving, growing, searching, and appreciating. It is about love and being in awe of beautiful things. We are able to distinguish between beauty and not beauty, and constructive and destructive things. For that reason, tai chi principles should be the philosophy of life and the practice of everyone. This will give people a better and more constructive life on earth. We will be spiraling upwards and harmonizing to higher and higher levels of human happiness.

In this world there are too many negative philosophies and restrictions. Too many laws inhibiting us. Do tai chi and just "let it be," *wu wei*, and seemingly do nothing yet accomplish everything. This is the beauty of tai chi.

The body and mind need the correct kind of stimulation. When you overcome any level of adversity, there will be a new level of achievement. It's a shame few people study tai chi or even just take an interest in something other than making money or buying things. I remember a Chinese intellectual saying about certain people, "They just eat and drink all day and don't use the mind. What a waste!" As I mention in *Chu Meditation*, a high level Taoist is called *Jung Yun*, a "real person." A real person will do the right, real things a person is supposed to do. Such a person is not phony, artificial, or acting. For that reason, we cannot find too many *Jung Yun* in this world.

### Tai Chi is a Counterweight to Nihilism

Tai Chi philosophy is constructive, healthy, and full of growth. It is the opposite of the negative, nay-saying, apocalyptic thinking of the West. Obsession with so-called "original sin," confessions and repenting is childish. People think we have all been condemned before we even do anything. That's how children are ruined. This power structure wants you kept off-balance and thinking you are full of sin and not worthy of anything. This makes it easier for organized religion and organized government to exploit you.

Too much negative thinking, nihilism, and stress, I believe, is a cause of cancer. Humans should not be gladiators fighting each other for the rest of us to watch and cheer. If each person extended a helping hand to everybody else, the world would be a better place. Helping each other is so much better than condoning aggressiveness and competitiveness, "mine versus yours" and "me versus them." We are part of the universe, part of the earth, like the flowers that bloom, the wind, the water and mountains. Beauty is just there. Nature can be surprisingly beautiful. Even the worst thunderstorm is part of nature and is beautiful because it can give rise to fresh air and more living things. A thunderstorm is a different variety of beauty, but it is still beautiful, depending on the way you look at it. The tai chi way of perceiving will change your life. Hopefully this book will inspire you to do tai chi correctly and the flame of tai chi's torch will never die.

## JUST DO IT

Just do the exercises. Everything will fall into place. Your body will tell you what is good for you. You don't make yourself, you are born a certain way — but you can use tai chi to improve what you have.

Just remember, tai chi is a treasure of body and mind. I think you are now ready to pursue it.

# GLOSSARY

**For Chinese characters and more words see the glossary in *TCCP&P*.**

*alignment:* a comprehensive descriptive term for the state of the whole body; it is the optimal relationship between cells, organs, bones, tendons, and muscles (etc.). Human bodies have an optimal composite but congenital problems or daily life can disrupt the relationship between the body's various parts causing pain and disease. Tai Chi training improves this relationship and that improvement facilitates *chi* circulation. A body in perfect health would have perfect alignment (see question 2.7). Alignment is also used to describe a posture or move. Brush Knee & Twist Step, for example, require the body to assume a particular internal relation with itself in order to be 'effective' or correct. This ideal position is also an alignment. Alignment, most often, is used as a short-hand for the ultimate goal of the tai chi practitioner: to make his or her body the best it can be to express his or her Tao (see questions 4.10, 4.12).

*approximation:* a pedagogical tool for teaching the form, as well as proper study habits. At first, students are taught the basic choreography of the moves broken down into smaller steps, executed mechanically. As the student masters these smaller steps, corrections can occur that refine the student's execution. The idea is that as the student learns to execute the form slowly, the body steadily improves its alignment, and an appreciation for the form's complexity dawns on the student. The more one trains, the more one can apply tai chi principles and the closer one gets to correct execution of the form, and not a distant approximation (see questions 4.4, 4.5, 4.6, 4.7).

*chi:* an electromagnetic force present in all living things, the 'life force' (see questions 2.4, 2.19 as well as *TCCP&P*, pp. 16-17).

*chi kung:* an exercise regimen that increases the amount of *chi* in the body. The regimen also improves *chi* circulation though a series of exercises coordinating proper body alignment and deep breathing (see chapter 6).

*chi vacuum:* is a term C. K. Chu uses to describe the condition that is created when doing *nei kung*. When you have a *chi* vacuum, the surrounding *chi* will rush into it, thus generating more *chi* (see *The Book of Nei Kung*, p.18).

*i:* mind power (see questions 3.3, 3.26 as well at *TCCP&P,* pp. 8, 14, 97-98).

*focusing:* as with an old-fashioned camera you must calculate correctly so that you are not too close or too far from your subject, and similarly you must correctly judge the distance between you and your opponent in order to deliver a powerful strike. (see 3.29).

*jou (yao):* soft, pliable, flexible like the movement of a whip or a snake. (see 1.4).

*kung fu:* Though this term has become colloquial for martial arts, it actually means a state of mastery. Thus, a master carpenter has 'kung fu,' meaning he does his task expertly and often performs beyond the range of simple description. The carpenter doesn't follow directions blindly but he feels his way through the materials to bring out the best qualities in the wood.

*li:* localized muscle strength (see question 3.3, as well at *TCCP&P,* p. 8).

*meridian:* the pathway *chi* follows as it circulates throughout the body (see question 2.19).

*nei kung* (sometimes spelled nei gong, nei gung): is a set of exercise that will generate a greater quantity of *chi* than regular *chi kung*. It works on the cellular level including the bones, tendons, organs, and muscles covering the whole body. Thus, it has the ability to firm the muscles and tendons. As a result of this training, the body will be extremely strong, yet pliable, and capable of withstanding the force of an opponent's attack. Higher level *nei kung* is called 'iron vest,' 'iron shirt' or 'golden bell system' because the body develops a 'muscle shield' that is very strong (see chapter 6).

Nei Kung: refers to the exercise system introduced in C. K. Chu's *The Book of Nei Kung. The Book of Nei Kung* was the first publication to give instructions in *nei kung* — in any language (see chapter 6 as well as *The Book of Nei Kung*).

*nei kung power:* the net effect of the body being in good health; the bones, tendons and muscles are aligned; the organs are working optimally; the mind is clear, calm, and relaxed (see 3.8, 6.22)

*pinyin*: Shorthand for *Hanyu Pinyin* (literally, 'Chinese language phonetics'), *pinyin* is the Romanization of Chinese approved of by the Chinese government in 1958. It became standard in 1979, replacing the Wade-Giles system of Romanization that went into effect in the mid-nineteenth century. As stated in the Note at the top of this text, in-house style of CK Chu Tai Chi is Wade Giles with a little pinyin as that was the style developed for the publication of *Tai Chi Chuan Principles & Practice* (1981).

*Push-Hands:* a two-person drill that serves as the basis for the application of tai chi movements to real fighting situations. The drill trains sensitivity, attacking, and yielding (see questions 5.22, 5.23).

*root:* positioning of the body so that it is like a tree, immovable (see questions 3.9, 3.20).

*Shaolin:* the external arts as promulgated by the monks of the Shaolin Temple. Like the Wu-tang system, it is a geographical term, too.

*tai chi principles:* a set of rules compiled by the old masters that must be observed in order to correctly move in the tai chi way (see questions 1.9, 2.24, 3.17, 4.11, 5.3).

*Tai Chi classics:* a set of works, mostly poetry and dialog, by old masters in which the tai chi principles are discussed (see question 1.9).

*Tai Chi Chuan:* the fighting system applying Taoist principles with health benefits. It is the soft internal martial art but there are several styles, such as Chen, Sun, Wu, and Yang (see Chapter 1).

*tai chi form:* A set choreography of movements based on Chang San-feng's original 13 movements that serve as the basic exercise formula for practitioners of tai chi. The number of movements varies with the style (see Introduction).

*tan tien:* shorthand for the lower *tan tien*, it is the energy center of the body and the functional center of the waist. It is located roughly an inch or two below the navel, whence all tai chi movement should originate. It is also a *chi* reservoir (see questions 2.20, 3.27, 4.9, 5.15, 5.26, 6.5, 6.17, 7.13).

*Tao:* means the path. And sometimes it means the only path. And for that reason it is like a law —. like the law of gravity. Moreover, each person has a Tao or 'a true nature' unique to that person, (see questions 1.5, 9.7)

*Taoism:* a study of the Tao. Through this study we try to get a better understanding of the inner mechanisms of nature, of the universe and of ourselves (see questions 1.5, 4.15, 9.11).

*waist:* The region of the human body between the pelvis and the rib cage. Tai chi movements come from the waist, specifically from the tan tien which is the center of the waist (see questions 5.3, 5.15, 5.18 and *TCCP&P, p.* 160)

*wushu* (or *wu shu*): the generic term for Chinese martial arts.

*Wu-tang system:* another name for tai chi chuan because Chang San-Feng, its creator, resided on Wu-tang (also Wudang) Mountain. Later, many other martial arts sprung up from this region. In general, the Wu-tang system is associated with internal arts while Shaolin Temple is associated with external systems.

*wu wei*: is to do something you like to do —without an artificial agenda. Most writers, following one another, interpret this term as "to do nothing".

*yielding*: a basic principle of tai chi fighting in which the fighter moves so as to minimize the opponent's action so there will be little reaction on his part; "bend to the opponent so that his strike doesn't find resistance, something to push against" (see questions 1.3, 1.8, 3.7, 3.10, 3.11, 3.16, 3.20, 5.5).

THIS BOOK WAS MADE POSSIBLE
BY A GENEROUS FINANCIAL
CONTRIBUTION FROM THE FOLLOWING:

### Platinum Level
Dan Nash
Dan Zegibe

### Jade Level
Cynthia Unterberg

### Gold Level
Caroline Chinlund
Sean O'Donohue
Grace Kim

### Silver Level
Roger Alexander
Martin Andrews
Richard Backer
Renae Edge
Norman Ellis
Michiko Kelly
Ahovi Kponou
John Lake
Ron Rice
Adam Rothenberg
Lee Velta

### Bronze Level
Miranda Cassel
Sarah Heggie
James Hicks
David I. Karabell
Dan Lawren
William Ngal
Joyce Pimble